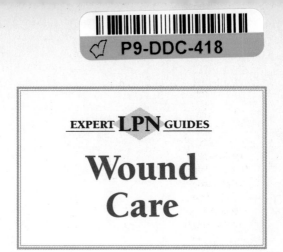

EXPERT **LPN** GUIDES

Wound
Care

EXPERT **LPN** GUIDES

Wound
Care

Wolters Kluwer | Lippincott Williams & Wilkins
Health

Philadelphia · Baltimore · New York · London
Buenos Aires · Hong Kong · Sydney · Tokyo

STAFF

EXECUTIVE PUBLISHER
Judith A. Schilling McCann, RN, MSN

EDITORIAL DIRECTOR
H. Nancy Holmes

CLINICAL DIRECTOR
Joan M. Robinson, RN, MSN

SENIOR ART DIRECTOR
Elaine Kasmer

CLINICAL MANAGER
Collette Bishop Hendler, RN, BS, CCRN

EDITORIAL PROJECT MANAGER
Christiane L. Brownell, ELS

CLINICAL PROJECT MANAGER
Kate Stout, RN, MSN, CCRN

EDITOR
Patricia Nale

COPY EDITORS
Kimberly Bilotta (supervisor),
Jen Fielding, Dorothy P. Terry,
Pamela Wingrod

DIGITAL COMPOSITION SERVICES
Diane Paluba (manager), Joyce Rossi
Biletz, Donald G. Knauss (project
manager)

MANUFACTURING
Beth J. Welsh

EDITORIAL ASSISTANTS
Megan L. Aldinger,
Karen J. Kirk, Linda K. Ruhf

INDEXER
Dianne Schneider

LPNWOUND010307

Library of Congress Cataloging-in-Publication Data

LPN expert guides. Wound care.
p. ; cm.
Includes bibliographical references and
index.
ISBN-13: 978-1-58255-702-1 (alk. paper)
ISBN-10: 1-58255-702-0 (alk. paper)
1. Wound healing—Handbooks, manuals,
etc. 2. Wounds and injuries—Nursing—
Handbooks, manuals, etc. 3. Wounds and
injuries—Treatment—Handbooks, manuals,
etc. I. Lippincott Williams & Wilkins. II.
Title: Wound care.
[DNLM: 1. Wounds and Injuries—nursing—Handbooks. 2. Nursing, Practical—
methods—Handbooks. WY 49 L9249
2007]
RD95.L556 2007
617.1--dc22   2006101491

Contents

Constitutional Brinksmanship

Contributors and consultants

Penny S. Bennett, RN, BSN
Charge Nurse Surgical Unit
Good Shepherd Health System
Longview, Tex.

KATHY COCHRAN, RN, MSN
Director of Practical Nursing
Department Chair for Health Technologies
Coosa Valley Technical College
Rome, Ga.

Dolores Cotton, RN, BSN, MS
Practical Nursing Coordinator
Meridian Technology Center
Stillwater, Okla.

Nancy Glassgow, RN, BSN
Nursing Instructor
Western Dakota Technical Institute
Rapid City, S.Dak.

Dustin Hicks, RN, BSN
Practical Nursing Instructor
Meridian Technology Center
Stillwater, Okla.

Roxanne Leisky, MSN, FNP, CWS
Owner
Advanced Wound Care, LLC
Springfield, Ill.

Patricia B. Lisk, RN, BSN
Instructor, Department Chair for CNA
Augusta (Ga.) Technical College

Kendra S. Seiler, RN, MSN
Nursing Instructor
Rio Hondo Community College
Whittier, Calif.

Gina Sirach, RN, MSN
Nursing Faculty
Southeastern Illinois College
Harrisburg

Laura Travis, RN, BSN
Health Careers Coordinator
Tennessee Technology Center at Dickson

WOUND CARE FUNDAMENTALS

Skin basics

The skin, or *integumentary system,* is the largest organ of the body. It accounts for 6 to 8 lb (2.5 to 3.5 kg) of a patient's body weight and has a surface area of more than 20 square feet. The thickest skin is located on the palms and on the soles; the thinnest skin, around the eyes and over the tympanic membranes in the ears.

Skin is made up of distinct layers that function as a single unit. The outermost layer, which is actually a layer of dead cells, is completely replaced every 4 to 6 weeks by cells that migrate to the surface from the layers beneath. The living cells in the skin receive oxygen and nutrients through an extensive network of small blood vessels. In fact, every square inch of skin contains more than 15′ blood vessels.

Skin protects the body by acting as a barrier between internal structures and the external world. Skin also stands between each of us and the social world around us, so it's no wonder that the condition and characteristics of a patient's skin influence how he feels about himself. When a patient has healthy skin—unblemished skin with good tone (firmness) and color—he feels better about himself.

Skin also reflects the general physical health of the body. For example, if blood oxygen levels are low, skin may look bluish; skin appears flushed or red when a patient has a fever.

Skin anatomy and physiology

Skin has two main layers: the epidermis and dermis. A layer of subcutaneous fatty connective tissue, sometimes called the *hypodermis,* lies beneath these layers. (See *A close look at skin.*)

Within the epidermis and dermis, which function as one interrelated unit, are five structural networks:
■ collagen fibers
■ elastic fibers
■ small blood vessels
■ nerve fibrils
■ lymphatics.

These networks are stabilized by hair and sweat gland ducts.

EPIDERMIS

The epidermis is the outermost of the skin's two main layers. It varies in thickness from about 0.004 inch (0.1 mm) thick on the eyelids to as much as 0.04 inch (1 mm) thick on the palms and soles. The epidermis is slightly acidic, with an average pH of 5.5. Covering the epidermis is the keratinized epithelium, a layer of cells that migrate up from the underlying dermis and die when they reach the surface. These cells are continuously generated and re-placed. The keratinized epithelium is supported by the dermis and underlying connective tissue.

The epidermis also contains *melanocytes* (cells that produce the brown pigment melanin), which give skin and hair their color. The more melanin produced by

A close look at skin

Major components of skin are the epidermis, dermis, and epidermal appendages.

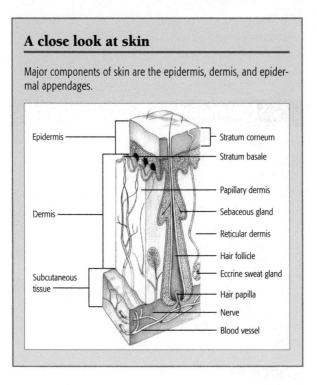

Epidermis
- Stratum corneum
- Stratum basale

Dermis
- Papillary dermis
- Sebaceous gland
- Reticular dermis
- Hair follicle

Subcutaneous tissue
- Eccrine sweat gland
- Hair papilla
- Nerve
- Blood vessel

melanocytes, the darker the skin. Skin color varies from one patient to the next, but it can also vary from one area of skin on the body to another. The hypothalamus regulates melanin production by secreting melanocyte-stimulating hormone.

The epidermis is divided into five distinct layers. Each layer's name reflects either its structure or its function. Let's look at them from the outside in:

■ The *stratum corneum* (horny layer) is the superficial layer of dead skin cells—the skin layer that's in contact with the environment. It has an acid mantle that helps protect the body from some fungi and bacteria. Cells in this layer are shed daily and replaced with cells from the layer beneath it. In such diseases as eczema and psoriasis, this layer may become abnormally thick and irritate skin structures and peripheral nerves.

■ The *stratum lucidum* (clear layer) is a single layer of cells that forms a transitional boundary between the stratum corneum above and the stratum granulosum below. This layer is most evident in areas where skin is thickest such as on the soles. It appears to be absent in areas where skin is especially thin such as on the eyelids. Although cells in this layer lack active nuclei, this is an area of intense enzyme activity that prepares cells for the stratum corneum.

■ The *stratum granulosum* (granular layer) is one to five cells thick and is characterized by flat cells with active nuclei. Experts believe this layer aids keratin formation.

■ The *stratum spinosum* (prickle-cell layer) is the area in which cells begin to flatten as they migrate toward the skin surface. Involucrin, a soluble protein precursor of the cornified envelopes of skin cells, is synthesized here.

■ The *stratum basale,* or stratum germinativum, is only one cell thick and is the only layer of the epidermis in which cells undergo mitosis to form new cells. The stratum basale forms the dermoepidermal junction— the area where the epidermis and dermis are connected. Protrusions of this layer (called *rete pegs* or *epidermal ridges*) extend down into the dermis where they're surrounded by vascularized dermal papillae. This unique structure supports the epidermis and facilitates the exchange of fluids and cells between the skin layers.

DERMIS

The dermis—the thick, deeper layer of skin—is composed of collagen and elastin fibers and an extracellular

Structural supports: Collagen and elastin

Normally, skin returns to its original position after it's pinched. This is because of the actions of the connective tissues collagen and elastin—two key components of skin.

UNDERSTANDING THE COMPONENTS

Collagen and elastin work together to support the dermis and give skin its physical characteristics.

COLLAGEN

Collagen fibers form tightly woven networks in the papillary layer of the dermis, or thick bundles paralleling the skin's surface. These fibers are relatively rigid and, therefore, give the dermis highly structured strength. In addition, collagen constitutes about 70% of the skin's dry weight and is its principal structural body protein.

ELASTIN

Elastin is composed of wavy fibers that intertwine with collagen in horizontal arrangements at the lower dermis and vertical arrangements at the epidermal margin. Elastin is the structural protein that allows stretch in the dermis.

SEEING THE EFFECTS OF AGE

As a person ages, collagen and elastin fibers break down, and the fine lines and wrinkles that are associated with aging develop. Extensive exposure to sunlight accelerates this breakdown process. Deep wrinkles are caused by changes in facial muscles. Over time, laughing, crying, smiling, and frowning cause facial muscles to thicken and eventually cause wrinkles in the overlying skin.

matrix, which contributes to skin's strength and pliability. Collagen fibers give skin its strength, and elastin fibers provide elasticity. The meshing of collagen and elastin determines the skin's physical characteristics. (See *Structural supports: Collagen and elastin.*) It's commonly called the *true skin.*

In addition, the dermis contains:

■ blood vessels and lymphatic vessels, which transport oxygen and nutrients to cells and remove waste products

■ nerve fibers and hair follicles, which contribute to skin sensation, temperature regulation, and excretion and absorption through the skin

■ fibroblast cells, which are important in the production of collagen and elastin.

The dermis is composed of two layers of connective tissue:

■ The papillary dermis, the outermost layer, is composed of collagen and reticular fibers, which are important in healing wounds. Capillaries in the papillary dermis carry the nourishment needed for metabolic activity.

■ The reticular dermis is the innermost layer. It's formed by thick networks of collagen bundles that anchor it to the subcutaneous tissue and underlying supporting structures, such as fasciae, muscle, and bone.

SEBACEOUS AND SUDORIFEROUS GLANDS

Although sebaceous and sudoriferous (or sweat) glands appear to originate in the dermis, they're actually appendages of the epidermis that extend downward into the dermis.

Sebaceous glands, found primarily in the skin of the scalp, face, upper body, and genital region, are part of the same structure that contains hair follicles. These saclike glands produce sebum, a fatty substance that lubricates and softens the skin. They are commonly referred to as *oil glands*.

Sweat glands are tightly coiled tubular glands; the average patient has roughly 2.6 million of them. They're present throughout the body in varying amounts: the palms and soles have many but the external ear, lip margins, nail beds, and glans penis have none.

The secreting portion of the sweat gland originates in the dermis and the outlet is on the surface of the skin. The sympathetic nervous system regulates the production of sweat, which, in turn, helps control body temperature.

There are two types of sweat glands:
■ eccrine
■ apocrine.

Eccrine glands are active at birth and are found throughout the body. They're most dense on the palms, soles, and forehead. These glands connect to the skin's surface through pores and produce sweat that lacks proteins and fatty acids. Eccrine glands are smaller than apocrine glands.

Apocrine glands begin to function at puberty. These glands open into hair follicles; therefore, most are found in areas where hair typically grows, such as the scalp, groin, and axillary region. The coiled secreting portion of the gland lies deep in the dermis (deeper than eccrine glands), and a duct connects it to the upper portion of the hair follicle. The sweat produced by apocrine glands contains the same water, sodium, and chloride produced by the eccrine glands, but it also contains proteins and fatty acids. It's thicker than the sweat produced by eccrine glands and has a milky-white or yellowish tinge. The unpleasant odor associated with sweat comes from the interaction of bacteria with these proteins and fatty acids.

SUBCUTANEOUS TISSUE

Subcutaneous tissue, or hypodermis, is a subdermal (below the skin) layer of loose connective tissue that contains major blood vessels, lymph vessels, and nerves. Subcutaneous tissue:
■ has a high proportion of fat cells and contains fewer small blood vessels than the dermis

- varies in thickness, depending on body type and location
- constitutes 15% to 20% of a man's weight and 20% to 25% of a woman's weight
- insulates the body
- absorbs shocks to the skeletal system
- helps skin move easily over underlying structures.

BLOOD SUPPLY

The skin receives its blood supply through vessels that originate in the underlying muscle tissue. Here, arteries branch into smaller vessels, which then branch into the network of capillaries that permeate the dermis and subcutaneous tissue.

Within the vascular system, only capillaries have walls thin enough (typically only a single layer of endothelial cells) to let solutes pass through. These thin walls allow nutrients and oxygen to pass from the bloodstream into the interstitial space around skin cells. At the same time, waste products pass into the capillaries and are carried away. The pressure of arterial blood entering the capillaries is about 30 mm Hg. The pressure of venous blood leaving the capillaries is about 10 mm Hg. (See *Fluid movement through capillary walls.*)

LYMPHATIC SYSTEM

The skin's lymphatic system helps remove waste products from the dermis.

Lymphatic vessels, or *lymphatics* for short, are similar to capillaries in that they're thin-walled, permeable vessels. However, lymphatics aren't part of the blood circulatory system. Instead, the lymphatics belong to a separate system that removes proteins, large waste products, and excess fluids from the interstitial spaces in skin and then transports them to the venous circulation. The lymphatics

Fluid movement through capillary walls

The movement of fluids through capillaries—a process called *capillary filtration*—results from blood pushing against the capillary walls. That pressure, called *hydrostatic* or *fluid-pushing* pressure, forces fluids and solutes through the capillary wall.

When the hydrostatic pressure inside a capillary is greater than the pressure in the surrounding interstitial space, fluids and solutes inside the capillary are forced out into the interstitial space, as shown here. When the pressure inside the capillary is less than the pressure outside, fluids and solutes move back in.

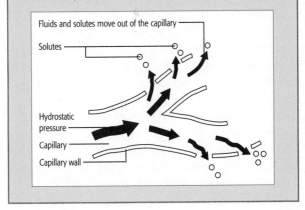

merge into two main trunks—the thoracic duct and the right lymphatic duct—which empty into the junction of the subclavian and internal jugular veins.

Functions of the skin

Skin performs, or participates in, a host of vital functions, including:

■ protection of internal structures

■ sensory perception

- thermoregulation
- excretion
- metabolism
- absorption
- social communication.

Damage to skin impairs its ability to perform these important functions.

PROTECTION

Skin acts as a physical and chemical barrier that protects the underlying tissue from mechanical injury and infection:

- Skin contains resident bacteria, which live on the skin and help provide resistance to pathogenic microorganisms and foreign matter by bacterial interference.
- Skin protects underlying tissue and structures from mechanical injury. Consider the feet for a moment. As a patient walks or runs, the soles of the feet withstand a tremendous amount of force, yet the underlying tissue and bone structures remain unharmed.
- Skin helps maintain a stable environment inside the body by preventing the loss of water, electrolytes, proteins, and other substances. Any damage—any wound—jeopardizes this protection. However, when damaged, skin goes into repair mode to restore full protection by stepping up the normal process of cell replacement.

SENSORY PERCEPTION

Nerve endings in the skin allow a patient to literally touch the world. Sensory nerve fibers originate in the nerve roots along the spine and supply specific areas of the skin known as *dermatomes*. Dermatomes document sensory function. This same network helps a patient avoid injury by making him aware of:

■ pain
■ pressure
■ heat
■ cold.

Sensory nerves exist throughout the skin; however, some areas are more sensitive than others—for example, the fingertips are more sensitive than the back. Sensation allows us to identify risks and avoid injury. Any loss or reduction of sensation—local or general—increases the chance of injury.

THERMOREGULATION

Thermoregulation, or control of body temperature, involves the concerted effort of nerves, blood vessels, and eccrine glands in the dermis:

■ When skin is exposed to cold or internal body temperature falls, blood vessels constrict, reducing blood flow and thereby conserving body heat.
■ When skin becomes too hot or internal body temperature rises, small arteries within the skin dilate, increasing the blood flow and sweat production to promote cooling.

EXCRETION

Unlikely as it may seem at first, the skin is an excretory organ. Excretion through the skin plays an important role in thermoregulation, electrolyte balance, and hydration. In addition, sebum excretion helps maintain the skin's integrity and suppleness.

Through its more than 2 million pores, skin efficiently transmits trace amounts of water and body wastes to the environment. At the same time, it prevents dehydration by ensuring that the body doesn't lose too much water.

Sweat carries water and salt to the skin surface where it evaporates, aiding thermoregulation and electrolyte balance. In addition, a small amount of water evaporates directly from the skin itself each day. A normal adult loses about 17 oz (500 ml) of water per day this way. While the skin is busy regulating fluids that are leaving the body, it's equally busy preventing unwanted or dangerous fluids from entering the body.

METABOLISM

Skin helps maintain the mineralization of bones and teeth. A photochemical reaction in the skin produces vitamin D, which is crucial to the metabolism of calcium and phosphate. These minerals, in turn, play a central role in the health of bones and teeth.

When skin is exposed to sunlight—that is, the ultraviolet (UV) spectrum in sunlight—vitamin D is synthesized in a photochemical reaction. Keep in mind, however, that overexposure to UV light causes skin damage that reduces the skin's ability to function properly.

ABSORPTION

Some drugs (and some toxic substances—pesticides, for example) can be absorbed directly through the skin and into the bloodstream. This process has been used to treat certain disorders via transdermal (skin patch) drug delivery systems. One of the best-known examples of this is the nicotine patch used in some smoking-cessation programs. This technology is also used to administer other medications, including forms of hormone replacement therapy, nitroglycerin, and some pain medications.

SOCIAL COMMUNICATION

A commonly overlooked but important function of the skin is its role in self-esteem development and social communication. Every time a patient looks in the mirror, he decides whether he likes what he sees. Although bone structure, body type, teeth, and hair (or lack thereof) all have an impact on a patient's self-esteem, the condition and characteristics of skin can have the greatest impact. Ask any teenager with acne. If a patient likes what he sees, self-esteem rises; if he doesn't, it sags.

Virtually every interpersonal exchange includes the nonverbal languages of facial expression and body posture. Level of self-esteem and skin characteristics—which are always visible—have an impact on how a patient communicates, both verbally and nonverbally, and how a listener receives the communication.

Because the physical characteristics of skin are so closely linked to self-perception, there has been a proliferation of skin care products and surgical techniques offered to keep skin looking young and healthy.

Aging and skin function

Over time, skin loses its ability to function as efficiently or as effectively as it once did. (See *How skin ages,* page 14.)

As a result, the golden years of life place a patient at greater risk for such injuries as pressure ulcers and tumors as well as various other skin conditions.

Although the entire body changes a great deal over time, several important changes in the skin increase the risk of wounds as a patient ages. These include:
▪ a 50% reduction in the cell turnover rate in the stratum corneum (outermost layer) and a 20% reduction in dermal thickness
▪ generalized reduction in dermal vascularization and an associated drop in blood flow to the skin

How skin ages

This table lists skin changes that normally occur with aging.

CHANGE	FINDINGS IN ELDERLY PATIENTS
Pigmentation	• Pale color
Thickness	• Wrinkling, especially on the face, arms, and legs • Parchmentlike appearance, especially over bony prominences and on the dorsal surfaces of the hands, feet, arms, and legs • Decreased fatty layers, providing less protection
Moisture	• Dry, flaky, and rough skin
Turgor	• "Tenting" of skin (skin standing alone)
Texture	• Numerous creases and lines

- redistribution of subcutaneous tissue, which contains fewer fat cells in elderly patients, to the stomach and thighs
- flattening of papillae in the dermoepidermal junction (meeting of the epidermis and dermis), which reduces adhesion between layers
- a drop in the number of Langerhans' cells (immune macrophages that attack invading germs) present in the skin
- a 50% decline in the number of fibroblasts and mast cells (cells that play a key role in the inflammatory response)
- a marked reduction in the ability to sense pressure, heat, and cold, although the same number of nerve endings in the skin are retained
- a significant decline in the number of sweat glands
- poorer absorption through the skin

■ a reduction in the skin's ability to synthesize vitamin D.

As a patient ages, physiologic changes increase the risk of various injuries. For example, elderly patients:

■ bruise easier and are more susceptible to edema around wounds because of reduced skin vascularization

■ are more likely to suffer pressure and thermal (hot and cold) damage to the skin because of diminished sensation

■ have a higher incidence of ischemia (cell damage resulting from too little oxygen reaching cells) in compressed tissue because bony areas have less subcutaneous cushioning and decreased sensation, causing an elderly patient to be less sensitive to the discomfort of remaining in one position for too long

■ risk hyperthermia and hypothermia because of decreased subcutaneous tissue

■ have fewer sweat glands and, therefore, produce less sweat, which hinders thermoregulation and increases the risk of hyperthermia

■ have a higher risk of skin infection because thinner skin is a less effective barrier to germs and allergens and because the skin contains fewer Langerhans' cells to fight infection and fewer mast cells to mediate the inflammatory response

■ are slower to exhibit a sensitization response (redness, heat, discomfort) because of the reduction in Langerhans' cells, resulting in overuse of topical drugs and more severe allergic reactions (because signs aren't evident early on)

■ risk overdose of transdermal drugs when poor absorption prompts them to reapply the medication too often

■ have a much higher incidence of shear and tear injuries because of compromised skin layer adhesion and less flexible collagen

■ have a reduction in sensation that prevents them from noticing the discomfort associated with impending skin ulcers.

Wound basics

Any damage to the skin is considered a wound. Wounds can result from planned events such as surgery, accidents such as a fall from a bike, or exposure to the environment such as the damage caused by UV rays in sunlight. Tissue damage in wounds varies widely, from a superficial break in the epithelium to deep trauma that involves the muscle and bone.

A *clean* wound is a wound produced by surgery. A *dirty* wound is one that may contain bacteria or debris. Trauma typically produces dirty wounds. The rate of recovery is influenced by the extent and type of damage incurred as well as other intrinsic factors, such as the patient's circulation, nutrition, and hydration status. However, regardless of the cause of a wound, the healing process is much the same in all cases.

Understanding wound healing

TYPES OF WOUND HEALING

Wounds are also classified by the way the wound closes. A wound can close by primary, secondary, or tertiary intention.

Primary intention

Primary intention involves reepithelialization, in which the skin's outer layer grows closed. Cells grow in from the margins of the wound and out from epithelial cells lining the hair follicles and sweat glands.

Wounds that heal through primary intention are, most commonly, superficial wounds that involve only the epidermis and don't involve the loss of tissue—for example, a first-degree burn. However, a wound that has well-approximated edges (edges that can be pulled together to meet neatly), such as a surgical incision, also heals through primary intention. Because there's no loss of tissue and little risk of infection, the healing process is predictable. These wounds usually heal in 4 to 14 days and result in minimal scarring.

Secondary intention

A wound that involves some degree of tissue loss heals by secondary intention. The edges of these wounds can't be easily approximated, and the wound itself is described as "partial thickness" or "full thickness," depending on its depth.

- Partial-thickness wounds extend through the epidermis and into, but not through, the dermis.
- Full-thickness wounds extend through the epidermis and dermis and may involve subcutaneous tissue, muscle and, possibly, bone.

During healing, wounds that heal by secondary intention fill with granulation tissue, a scar forms, and reepithelialization occurs, primarily from the wound edges. Pressure ulcers, second- and third-degree burns, dehisced surgical wounds, and traumatic injuries are examples of this type of wound. These wounds also take longer to heal, result in scarring, and have a higher rate of complications than wounds that heal by primary intention.

Tertiary intention

When a wound is intentionally kept open to allow edema or infection to resolve or to permit removal of exudate, the wound heals by tertiary intention, or delayed primary intention. The wound is then closed with sutures, staples, or adhesive skin closures. These wounds result in more scarring than wounds that heal by primary intention but less than those that heal by secondary intention.

PHASES OF WOUND HEALING

The healing process is the same for all wounds, whether the cause is mechanical, chemical, or thermal.

Health care professionals discuss the process of wound healing in four specific phases:

■ hemostasis
■ inflammation
■ proliferation
■ maturation.

Although this categorization is useful, it's important to remember that healing rarely occurs in this strict order. Typically, the phases of wound healing overlap. (See *How wounds heal.*)

Hemostasis

Immediately after an injury, the body releases chemical mediators and intercellular messengers called *growth factors* that begin the process of cleaning and healing the wound.

When blood vessels are damaged, the small muscles in the walls of the vessels contract (vasoconstriction), reducing the flow of blood to the injury and minimizing blood loss. Vasoconstriction can last as long as 30 minutes.

Next, blood leaking from the inflamed, dilated, or broken vessels begins to coagulate. Collagen fibers in the

SPOTLIGHT

How wounds heal

The healing process begins at the instant of injury and proceeds through a repair cascade, as outlined here.

1. When tissue is damaged, serotonin, histamine, prostaglandins, and blood from the injured vessels fill the area. Blood platelets form a clot, and fibrin in the clot binds the wound edges together.

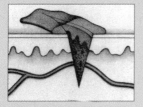

2. Lymphocytes start the inflammatory response, increasing capillary permeability. Wound edges swell; white blood cells from surrounding vessels move in and ingest bacteria and cellular debris, demolishing the clot. Redness, warmth, swelling, pain, and loss of function may occur.

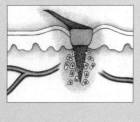

3. Adjacent healthy tissue supplies blood, nutrients, fibroblasts, proteins, and other building materials needed to form soft, pink, and highly vascular granulation tissue, which begins to bridge the area. Inflammation may decrease, or signs and symptoms of infection (increased swelling, increased pain, fever, and pus-filled discharge) may develop.

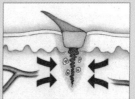

4. Fibroblasts in the granulation tissue secrete collagen, a gluelike substance. Collagen fibers crisscross the area, forming scar tissue.

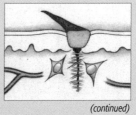

(continued)

How wounds heal *(continued)*

5. Meanwhile, epithelial cells at the wound edge multiply and migrate toward the wound center. A new layer of surface cells replaces the layer that was destroyed. New, healthy tissue or granulation tissue (if the blood supply is inadequate) appears.

6. Damaged tissue (including lymphatics, blood vessels, and stromal matrices) regenerates. Collagen fibers shorten, and the scar gets smaller. The size of the scar may continue to decrease and normal function return or the scar may hypertrophy, leading to the formation of a keloid and the development of contractures.

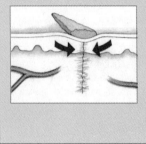

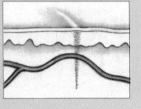

wall of the damaged blood vessels activate the platelets in the blood in the wound. Aided by the action of prostaglandins, the platelets enlarge and stick together to form a temporary plug in the blood vessel, which helps prevent further bleeding. The platelets also release additional vasoconstrictors—such as serotonin—which help prevent further blood loss. Thrombin forms in a cascade of events stimulated by the platelets, and a clot forms to close the small vessels and stop bleeding.

This initial phase of wound healing occurs almost immediately after the injury occurs and works quickly (within minutes) in small wounds. It's less effective in stopping the bleeding in larger wounds.

Inflammation

The inflammatory phase is both a defense mechanism and a crucial component of the healing process. (See *Understanding the inflammatory response*, page 22.)

During this phase, the wound is cleaned and the process of rebuilding begins. This phase is marked by swelling, redness, and heat at the wound site.

During the inflammatory phase, vascular permeability increases, permitting serous fluid carrying small amounts of cell and plasma protein to accumulate in the tissue around the wound (edema). The accumulation of fluid causes the damaged tissue to appear swollen, red, and warm to the touch.

During the early phase of the inflammatory process, *neutrophils* (a type of white blood cell) enter the wound. The primary role of neutrophils is phagocytosis, or the removal and destruction of bacteria and other contaminants.

As neutrophil infiltration slows, *monocytes* appear. Monocytes are converted into activated macrophages and continue the job of cleaning the wound. The macrophages play a key role early in the process of granulation and reepithelialization by producing growth factors and by attracting the cells needed for the formation of new blood vessels and collagen.

The inflammatory phase of healing is important for preventing wound infection. The process is negatively influenced if the patient has a systemic condition that suppresses his immune system or if he's undergoing immunosuppressive therapy. In clean wounds, the inflammatory response lasts about 36 hours. In dirty or infected wounds, the response can last much longer.

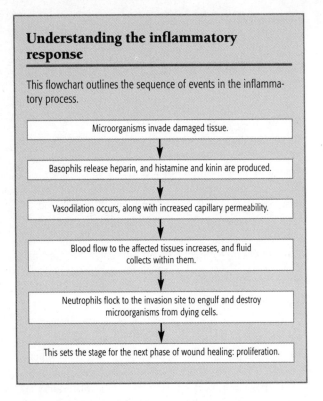

Understanding the inflammatory response

This flowchart outlines the sequence of events in the inflammatory process.

Microorganisms invade damaged tissue.

↓

Basophils release heparin, and histamine and kinin are produced.

↓

Vasodilation occurs, along with increased capillary permeability.

↓

Blood flow to the affected tissues increases, and fluid collects within them.

↓

Neutrophils flock to the invasion site to engulf and destroy microorganisms from dying cells.

↓

This sets the stage for the next phase of wound healing: proliferation.

Proliferation

During the proliferation phase of the healing process, the body:

- fills the wound with connective tissue (granulation)
- contracts the wound edges (contraction)
- covers the wound with epithelium (epithelialization).

All wounds go through the proliferation phase; it takes much longer, however, in wounds with extensive tissue loss. Although phases overlap, wound granulation generally starts when the inflammatory response is complete. As the inflammatory phase subsides, the wound exudate (drainage) begins to decrease.

The proliferation phase involves regeneration of blood vessels (angiogenesis) and the formation of connective or granulation tissue. The development of granulation tissue requires an adequate supply of blood and nutrients. Endothelial cells in blood vessels in surrounding tissue reconstruct damaged or destroyed vessels by first migrating and then proliferating to form new capillary beds. As the beds form, this area of the wound takes on a red, granular (also called *beefy*) appearance. This tissue is a good defense against contaminants, but it's also quite fragile and bleeds easily.

During the proliferation phase, growth factors prompt fibroblasts to migrate to the wound. Fibroblasts are the most common cell in connective tissue; they're responsible for making fibers and ground substance, also known as *extracellular matrix*, which provides support to cells. At first, fibroblasts populate just the margins of the wound; they later spread over the entire wound surface.

Fibroblasts have the important task of synthesizing collagen fibers that, in turn, produce keratinocyte—a growth factor needed for reepithelialization. This process necessitates a delicate balance of collagen synthesis and lysis (making new and removing old). If the process yields too much collagen, increased scarring results. If the process yields too little collagen, scar tissue is weak and easily ruptured. Because fibroblasts require a supply of oxygen to perform their important role, capillary bed regeneration is crucial to the process.

As healing progresses, myofibroblasts and the newly formed collagen fibers contract, pulling the wound edges toward each other. Contraction reduces the amount of granulation tissue needed to fill the wound, thereby

Contraction vs. contracture

Contraction and contracture occur during the wound-healing process. Although they have mechanisms in common, it's important to understand how contraction and contracture differ.

• *Contraction,* a desirable process that occurs during healing, is the process by which the edges of a wound pull toward the center of the wound to close it. Contraction continues to close the wound until tension in the surrounding skin causes it to slow and then stop.

• *Contracture* is an undesirable process and a common complication of burn scarring. Typically, contracture occurs after healing is complete. Contracture involves an inordinate amount of pulling or shortening of tissue, resulting in an area of tissue with a limited ability to move. It's especially problematic over joints, which may be pulled to a flexed position. Stretching is the only way to overcome contracture, and patients typically require physical therapy to help them accomplish this goal.

speeding the healing process. (See *Contraction vs. contracture.*) Complete healing occurs only after epithelial cells have completely covered the surface of the wound. As this occurs, keratinocytes switch from a migratory mode to a differentiative mode. The epidermis thickens and becomes differentiated, and the wound is closed. Any remaining scab comes off and the new epidermis is toughened by the production of keratin, which also returns the skin to its original color.

Maturation

The final phase of wound healing is maturation, which is marked by the shrinking and strengthening of the scar. This gradual, transitional phase of healing can continue for months, or even years, after the wound has closed.

During this phase, fibroblasts leave the site of the wound, vascularization is reduced, the scar shrinks and becomes pale, and the mature scar forms. If the wound involved destruction of extensive tissue, the scar won't contain hair, sweat, or sebaceous glands.

The wound gradually gains tensile strength. In primary intention wounds, tissues will achieve about 30% to 50% of their original strength between days 1 and 14. When fully healed, tissue will achieve, at best, about 80% of its original strength. Scar tissue will always be less elastic than the surrounding skin.

FACTORS THAT AFFECT HEALING

The healing process is affected by many factors. The most important influences are:

■ nutrition
■ oxygenation
■ infection
■ age
■ chronic health conditions
■ medications
■ smoking.

Nutrition

Proper nutrition is the most important factor affecting wound healing. Unfortunately, malnutrition is a common finding among patients with wounds; it's reported in 30% of adult surgical patients and 45% to 57% of nonsurgical patients. For elderly adults, the problem is more pervasive. Malnutrition is reported in 53% to 74% of elderly hospitalized patients.

Poor nutrition prolongs hospitalization and increases the risk of medical complications, with the severity of complications being directly related to the severity of the malnutrition. In elderly patients, malnutrition is known to

Tips for detecting nutritional problems

Nutritional problems may stem from physical conditions, drugs, diet, or lifestyle factors. This list can help you identify risk factors that make your patient particularly susceptible to nutritional problems.

PHYSICAL CONDITION
- Chronic illnesses such as diabetes and neurologic, cardiac, or thyroid problems
- Family history of diabetes or heart disease
- Draining wounds or fistulas
- Weight issues—weight loss of 5% of normal body weight; weight less than 90% of ideal body weight; weight gain or loss of 10 lb (4.5 kg) or more in last 6 months; obesity; or weight gain of 20% above normal body weight
- History of GI disturbances
- Anorexia or bulimia
- Depression or anxiety
- Severe trauma
- Recent chemotherapy or radiation therapy

- Physical limitations, such as paresis or paralysis
- Recent major surgery
- Pregnancy, especially teen or multiple-birth pregnancy

DRUGS AND DIET
- Fad diets
- Corticosteroid, diuretic, or antacid use
- Mouth, tooth, or denture problems
- Excessive alcohol intake
- Strict vegetarian diet
- Liquid diet or nothing by mouth for more than 3 days

LIFESTYLE FACTORS
- Lack of support from family or friends
- Financial problems

increase the risk of pressure ulcers and delay wound healing. It may also contribute to poor tensile strength in healing wounds and an associated increase in the risk of wound dehiscence. (See *Tips for detecting nutritional problems.*) Protein is critical for wounds to heal properly. In fact, a patient needs to double the recommended dietary allowance of protein (from 0.8 to 1.6 g/kg/day) before tissue even begins to heal. If a significant amount of body weight has been lost with the injury, as much as 50% of the lost weight must be regained before healing will begin. A patient who lacks protein reserves heals slowly, if at all, and a patient who's borderline malnourished can easily become malnourished under this demand.

The body needs protein to form collagen during the proliferation phase. Without adequate protein, collagen formation is reduced or delayed and the healing process is slowed. Studies of malnourished patients indicate that they have lower levels of serum albumin, which results in slower oxygen diffusion and, in turn, a reduction in the ability of neutrophils to kill bacteria. Wound exudate alone can contain up to 100 g of protein per day.

Fatty acids (lipids) are used in cell structures and play a role in the inflammatory process. Also, vitamins C, B-complex, A, and E and the minerals iron, copper, zinc, and calcium are important in the healing process. A zinc deficiency adversely affects the proliferation phase by slowing the rate of epithelialization and decreasing the strength of collagen produced—and, thus, the strength of the wound.

In addition to protein and zinc, collagen synthesis requires supplies of carbohydrates and fat. Collagen cross-linking requires adequate amounts of vitamins A and C, iron, and copper. Vitamin C, iron, and zinc are important to developing tensile strength during the maturation phase of wound healing.

Oxygenation

Healing depends on a regular supply of oxygen. For example, oxygen is critical for leukocytes to destroy bacteria and for fibroblasts to stimulate collagen synthesis. If the supply is hindered by poor blood flow to the area of the wound or if the patient's ability to take in adequate oxygen is impaired, the result is the same—impaired healing.

Possible causes of inadequate blood flow to the area of the wound include pressure, arterial occlusion, or prolonged vasoconstriction, possibly associated with such medical conditions as peripheral vascular disease and atherosclerosis. Possible causes of a lower than necessary systemic blood oxygenation include:

- inadequate oxygen intake
- hypothermia or hyperthermia
- anemia
- alkalemia (rise in blood pH)
- other medical conditions such as chronic obstructive pulmonary disease.

Infection

Infection can be systemic or localized in the wound. A systemic infection, such as pneumonia or tuberculosis, increases the patient's metabolism and thus consumes the fluids, nutrients, and oxygen that the body needs for healing.

A localized infection in the wound itself is more common. Remember, any break in the skin allows bacteria to enter. The infection may occur as part of the injury or may develop later in the healing process. For example, when the inflammatory phase lingers, wound healing is delayed and metabolic by-products of bacterial ingestion accumulate in the wound. This buildup interferes with the formation of new blood vessels and the synthesis of collagen. Infection can also occur in a wound that has been healing normally. This is especially true for larger wounds involving extensive tissue damage. New or increased pain, redness, heat, and drainage are signs of a new infection. In any case, healing can't progress until the cause of infection is addressed.

Effects of aging on wound healing

In older patients, these factors impede wound healing:

● poorer oxygenation at the wound because of increasingly fragile capillaries and a reduction in skin vascularization

● slower turnover rate in epidermal cells

● altered nutrition and fluid intake resulting from physical changes that can accompany aging, such as reduced saliva production, a declining sense of smell and taste, or decreased stomach motility

● altered nutrition and fluid intake attributable to troubling personal or social issues, such as loose-fitting dentures, financial concerns, eating alone after the death of a spouse, or problems preparing or obtaining food

● impaired function of the respiratory or immune systems

● reduced dermal and subcutaneous mass leading to an increased risk of chronic pressure ulcers

● healed wounds that lack skin strength and are susceptible to reinjury.

In many patients with chronic illnesses, infection may result from fecal contamination. Fecal incontinence affects 20% of chronically ill patients and is associated with increased mortality. Typically, those affected are patients with poorer overall health.

Age

Skin changes that occur with aging cause healing time to be prolonged in elderly patients. Although delayed healing is partially due to physiologic changes, it's usually complicated by other problems associated with aging, such as poor nutrition and hydration, the presence of a chronic condition, or the use of multiple medications. (See *Effects of aging on wound healing*.)

Chronic health conditions

Respiratory problems, atherosclerosis, diabetes, and malignancies can increase the risk of wounds and interfere with wound healing. These conditions can interfere with systemic and peripheral oxygenation and nutrition, which affect healing.

Impaired circulation, a common problem for patients with diabetes and other disorders, can cause tissue hypoxia (lack of oxygen). Neuropathy associated with diabetes reduces a patient's ability to sense pressure. As a result, a patient with diabetes may experience trauma, especially to the feet, without realizing it. Insulin dependency can impair leukocyte function, which adversely affects cell proliferation.

Hemiplegia and quadriplegia involve the breakdown of muscle tissue and reduction in the padding around the large bones of the lower body. Because a patient with one of these conditions lacks sensation, he's at risk for developing chronic pressure ulcers.

Normally, a healthy patient shifts position every 15 minutes or so, even during sleep. This prevents tissue damage due to ischemia. Anything that impairs the ability to sense pressure, including the use of pain medications, spinal cord lesions, or cognitive impairment, puts the patient at risk for pressure wounds (the patient can't feel the growing discomfort of pressure and respond to it).

Other conditions that can delay healing include:
- dehydration
- end-stage renal disease
- thyroid disease
- heart failure
- peripheral vascular disease
- vasculitis and other collagen vascular disorders.

Drugs

Any drug that reduces a patient's movement, circulation, or metabolic function, such as sedatives and tranquilizers, can inhibit the patient's ability to sense and respond to pressure. Also, because movement promotes adequate oxygenation, lack of motion means that peripheral blood delivers less oxygen to the extremities than it should. This is especially problematic for elderly adults. Remember, oxygen is important; without it, the healing process slows and the risk of complications increases.

Some medications, such as corticosteroids and chemotherapeutic drugs, reduce the body's ability to mount an appropriate inflammatory response. This interrupts the inflammatory phase of healing and can dramatically lengthen healing time, especially in patients with compromised immune systems such as those with acquired immunodeficiency syndrome.

Smoking

Carbon monoxide, a component of cigarette smoke, binds to the hemoglobin in blood in the place of oxygen. This significantly reduces the amount of oxygen circulating in the bloodstream, which can impede wound healing. To some extent, this reaction also occurs in people regularly exposed to second-hand smoke.

COMPLICATIONS OF WOUND HEALING

The most common complications associated with wound healing are hemorrhage, dehiscence and evisceration, infection, and fistula formation.

Hemorrhage

Internal hemorrhage (bleeding) can result in the formation of a hematoma—a blood clot that solidifies to form a

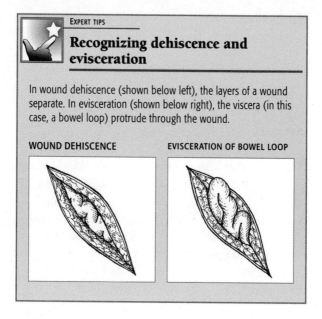

Recognizing dehiscence and evisceration

In wound dehiscence (shown below left), the layers of a wound separate. In evisceration (shown below right), the viscera (in this case, a bowel loop) protrude through the wound.

WOUND DEHISCENCE

EVISCERATION OF BOWEL LOOP

hard lump under the skin. Hematomas are commonly found around bruises.

External hemorrhage is visible bleeding from the wound. External bleeding during healing isn't unusual because the newly developed blood vessels are fragile and rupture easily. This is one reason a wound needs to be protected by a dressing. However, each time the new blood vessels suffer damage, healing is delayed while repairs are made.

Dehiscence and evisceration

Dehiscence is a separation of skin and tissue layers. It's most likely to occur 3 to 11 days after the injury was sustained and may follow surgery. Evisceration is similar but involves protrusion of underlying visceral organs as well. (See *Recognizing dehiscence and evisceration*.)

Dehiscence and evisceration may constitute a surgical emergency, especially if they involve an abdominal wound. If a wound opens without evisceration, it may need to heal by secondary intention. Poor nutrition, obesity, and advanced age are several factors that increase a patient's risk of dehiscence and evisceration.

Infection

Infection is a relatively common complication of wound healing that should be addressed promptly. Infection can lead to a cellulitis or bacterial infection that spreads to surrounding tissue. Signs that infection may be at work include:

- redness and warmth of the margins and tissue around the wound
- fever
- edema
- pain (or a sudden increase in pain)
- pus
- increase in exudate or a change in its color
- odor
- discoloration of granulation tissue
- further wound breakdown or lack of progress toward healing.

Fistula formation

A fistula is an abnormal passage between two organs or between an organ and the skin. In a wound, it may appear as undermining or a sinus tract in the skin around the wound. If a sinus tract (or tunneling) is present, it's important to determine its extent and direction.

2

NUTRITION IN WOUND CARE

Proper nutrition is an essential aspect of wound care. Poor nutrition can have many effects on the skin and healing process; therefore, it's critical to identify and treat existing malnutrition. There must be adequate levels of many nutrients for the healing process to occur, such as protein, calories, vitamins, and minerals. In addition, cells require adequate water to store and process nutrients.

To optimize nursing care of a patient with a wound, it's necessary to properly assess the patient's nutritional status to effectively plan and implement nursing strategies that enhance quality health. (See *Optimizing nutrition in a wound-care patient.*)

Laboratory test results

Laboratory test results can be useful in identifying the level of nutritional depletion and the expected rate of wound healing. Some important laboratory values in wound healing are discussed here.

TOTAL PROTEIN

Total protein is a cumulative measurement of all types of protein in the bloodstream. The normal range of protein is 6 to 8.5 g/dl. Lower levels of protein can lead to de-

Optimizing nutrition in a wound-care patient

Optimizing nutrition in a wound-care patient takes planning, assessment, and follow-up. Here are suggested interventions to help the wound-care patient obtain the required nutrition.

- Encourage high-calorie and high-protein foods.
- Allow friends and family members to bring in favorite foods.
- Liberalize diet restrictions as much as possible.
- Address issues with ill-fitting dentures; try different consistencies of food if the patient has difficulty chewing.
- Encourage adequate fluid intake as allowed.
- Use a protein supplement, as ordered, if the patient has a low albumin or prealbumin level.
- Monitor the patient's glucose level.
- If appropriately trained and per facility policy, administer a multivitamin and I.V. fluids if the patient can't take adequate oral fluid intake.
- If the patient can't meet his nutritional needs with oral intake alone, collaborate with the health care practitioner to consider enteral support.

creased antibody production and an increased risk of infection. Protein is also needed for collagen synthesis—an important aspect of wound healing and maintaining good skin turgor

ALBUMIN

Albumin, a visceral protein made in the liver, is a good indicator of the patient's protein status for the past 2 or 3 weeks. The normal range for albumin is 3.5 to 5 mg/dl, the level required for optimal healing. Mildly depleted albumin levels are 3 to 3.4 mg/dl; moderately depleted, 2.7 to 2.9 mg/dl; and severely depleted, 2.5 mg/dl and less. The more depleted the albumin level, the slower the recovery process.

PREALBUMIN

Prealbumin has a half-life of 2 or 3 days and is more responsive to acute changes in nutritional status. Wound healing is less likely to occur in patients with low prealbumin levels.

The normal range needed for optimal wound healing is 18 to 45 mg/dl. Mildly depleted levels of prealbumin are 10 to 17 mg/dl; moderately depleted levels, 5 to 10 mg/dl; and severely depleted, less than 5 mg/dl. The prealbumin level should be assessed every 3 days when changing the patient's nutritional intake. Prealbumin levels should improve 0.5 to 1 mg/dl per day to indicate a positive effective change in the patient's protein status.

GLUCOSE

It's important to monitor glucose levels in the wound-care patient because higher levels of glucose in the bloodstream can hinder the healing process at the capillary level. Even if the patient doesn't have diabetes, the glucose level needs to be monitored because certain medications such as corticosteroids can lead to elevated levels. The normal range for blood glucose is 70 to 130 mg/dl. Consistently higher levels can hinder the healing process. Other factors, such as infection, stress, and the patient's noncompliance with antidiabetic drugs can also increase the glucose level.

GLYCOSYLATED HEMOGLOBIN

Glycosylated hemoglobin (HbA_{1C}) is important to monitor in patients with diabetes because it indicates the patient's average glucose level for the previous 2 or 3 months. The normal range for HbA_{1C} is 4 to 6.7 mg/dl;

levels above 7 mg/dl indicate that the patient's blood glucose is poorly controlled.

NUTRITIONAL STATUS

To ensure that the healing process is most efficient and effective, it's critical to evaluate and treat the nutritional status of the wound-care patient. This process can help identify patients most at risk for poor healing so that prompt intervention can occur. The healing process can proceed only after the patient's nutritional deficiencies are corrected.

Physical signs of nutritional deficiency

These signs can indicate specific vitamin and mineral deficiencies (see *Evaluating nutritional disorders,* pages 38 and 39):

- hair loss
- brittle nails
- edema
- mouth sores
- swollen gums
- red, swollen tongue.

Provide the wound-care patient with a multivitamin and mineral supplement to ensure adequate micronutrient intake. Commercial nutritional supplements contain micronutrient supplementation, and all enteral formulas contain adequate levels of micronutrients. All foods consumed by the patient contribute to his overall daily intake of vitamins and minerals.

Evaluating nutritional disorders

This chart can help you interpret your nutritional assessment findings. Body systems are listed with signs or symptoms and the implications for each.

BODY SYSTEM OR REGION	SIGN OR SYMPTOM	IMPLICATIONS
GENERAL	• Weakness and fatigue	• Anemia or electrolyte imbalance
	• Weight loss	• Decreased calorie intake, increased calorie use, or inadequate nutrient intake or absorption
SKIN, HAIR, AND NAILS	• Dry, flaky skin	• Vitamin A, vitamin B-complex, or linoleic acid deficiency
	• Dry skin with poor turgor	• Dehydration
	• Rough, scaly skin with bumps	• Vitamin A deficiency
	• Petechiae or ecchymoses	• Vitamin C or K deficiency
	• Sore that won't heal	• Protein, vitamin C, or zinc deficiency
	• Thinning, dry hair	• Protein deficiency
	• Spoon-shaped, brittle, or ridged nails	• Iron deficiency
EYES	• Night blindness; corneal swelling, softening, or dryness; Bitot's spots (gray triangular patches on the conjunctiva)	• Vitamin A deficiency
	• Red conjunctiva	• Riboflavin deficiency

Evaluating nutritional disorders (continued)

BODY SYSTEM OR REGION	SIGN OR SYMPTOM	IMPLICATIONS
THROAT AND MOUTH	• Cracks at the corner of mouth	• Riboflavin or niacin deficiency
	• Magenta tongue	• Riboflavin deficiency
	• Beefy, red tongue	• Vitamin B_{12} deficiency
	• Soft, spongy, bleeding gums	• Vitamin C deficiency
	• Swollen neck (goiter)	• Iodine deficiency
CARDIOVASCULAR	• Edema	• Protein deficiency
	• Tachycardia, hypotension	• Dehydration
GASTROINTESTINAL	• Ascites	• Protein deficiency
MUSCULOSKELETAL	• Bone pain and bow leg	• Vitamin D or calcium deficiency
	• Muscle wasting	• Protein, carbohydrate, and fat deficiency
NEUROLOGIC	• Altered mental status	• Dehydration and thiamine or vitamin B_{12} deficiency
	• Paresthesia	• Vitamin B_{12}, pyridoxine, or thiamine deficiency

Body mass index

The body mass index (BMI) uses weight and height to help classify a person as underweight, normal, or obese. (See *Determining BMI*, page 40.) A BMI of less than 18 is considered underweight, 18.5 to 24.9 is normal weight, 25 to 29.9 is overweight, and 30 and above is obese. Patients whose BMI is 18 or less have the poorest nutritional status. A person can have a high BMI and still be protein

Determining BMI

Body mass index (BMI) measures weight in relation to height.
The BMI ranges shown here are for adults. They aren't exact
ranges for healthy or unhealthy weights; however, they show that
health risks increase at higher levels of overweight and obesity.
To use the graph, find your patient's weight along the bottom
and then go straight up until you come to the line that matches
his height. The shaded area indicates whether your patient is
healthy, overweight, or obese.

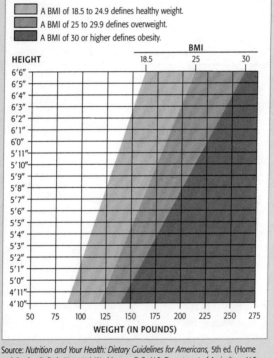

A BMI of 18.5 to 24.9 defines healthy weight.
A BMI of 25 to 29.9 defines overweight.
A BMI of 30 or higher defines obesity.

Source: *Nutrition and Your Health: Dietary Guidelines for Americans,* 5th ed. (Home
and Garden Bulletin No. 232.) Washington, D.C.: U.S. Department of Agriculture, U.S.
Department of Health and Human Services, 2000.

malnourished, however, if his food intake is high in fats and carbohydrates but isn't rich in proteins. To help identify this type of protein malnourishment, ask the patient to list his favorite foods.

WEIGHT HISTORY

Assess the patient for recent weight gain or loss. A significant weight loss is indicated when the patient has lost 10% of his body weight in 6 months, 5% of his body weight in 1 month, or 2% of his body weight in 1 week. Remember that weight gain doesn't necessarily indicate good nutritional status. Fluid retention because of edema, heart failure, or poor kidney function can contribute to significant weight gain that isn't body fat or muscle. Even if weight gain is due to a good appetite, it's the food type and its nutritional value that's important.

RECENT APPETITE

Assess the amount of food in the patient's current intake and observe him at mealtimes if possible. Assess whether the patient has diet restrictions related to disease or cultural or religious beliefs and practices. In addition, be sure to inquire about recent changes in appetite from his normal intake that may be attributed to lack of or poor-fitting dentures, mouth or tooth procedures, death of a loved one or pet, or financial concerns. Obtain a list of the drugs he's taking and ask if any have affected his taste. (See *Prescription drugs and anorexia*, page 42.) Many drug can affect a patient's taste, which can cause a decrease in appetite and result in a poor nutritional status.

The more factors present, the poorer the nutritional status. The longer the poor intake continues, the worse the nutritional status becomes. The longer a patient has a poor nutritional status, the longer the wound will take to heal. The patient first has to return to a normal nutrient

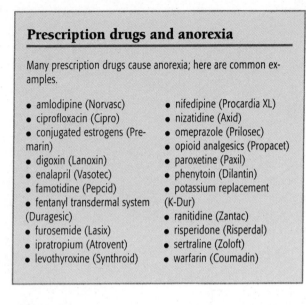

Prescription drugs and anorexia

Many prescription drugs cause anorexia; here are common examples.

- amlodipine (Norvasc)
- ciprofloxacin (Cipro)
- conjugated estrogens (Premarin)
- digoxin (Lanoxin)
- enalapril (Vasotec)
- famotidine (Pepcid)
- fentanyl transdermal system (Duragesic)
- furosemide (Lasix)
- ipratropium (Atrovent)
- levothyroxine (Synthroid)

- nifedipine (Procardia XL)
- nizatidine (Axid)
- omeprazole (Prilosec)
- opioid analgesics (Propacet)
- paroxetine (Paxil)
- phenytoin (Dilantin)
- potassium replacement (K-Dur)
- ranitidine (Zantac)
- risperidone (Risperdal)
- sertraline (Zoloft)
- warfarin (Coumadin)

intake before his calorie and protein intake can be supplemented and healing promoted.

PROTEIN STATUS

Assess the patient's protein status by obtaining the prealbumin, albumin, and total protein levels. Look for medications or other factors that may alter these values. Remember to review all laboratory values together and not to look at one value only.

The wound

The wound itself can indicate a patient's nutritional status. More complex wounds require more calories and protein to complete the healing process; therefore, the more complex the wound, the more potential for poor nutritional status. Multiple wounds also have a higher requirement for calories and protein to heal, so patients with multiple wounds are more likely to have a poorer nutritional status.

The longer a wound has been present, the more likely it is that the patient's lifestyle has been affected, which can lead to depression, pain, or lack of mobility. These factors can affect a patient's intake of essential nutrients and lead to poor nutritional status.

Nutritional guidelines

Consider these guidelines when determining a patient's nutritional needs. To optimize nutrition, a patient needs the right amount of:
■ calories
■ protein
■ fluid.

CALORIE NEEDS
Adequate calories are required to maintain body functions such as temperature regulation. Extra calories are required when the patient has a fever, infection, or a wound.

Calorie needs are typically best expressed in a range. If the patient stays within that range of calorie consumption on most days, then he's likely getting adequate calories. A prolonged decrease in calorie intake, however, can lead to poor nutritional status, poor wound healing, and weight loss.

There are many ways to calculate calorie needs depending on the available time and resources. (See *Determining calorie needs*, pages 44 and 45.)

It's important to remember that a wound is a stressor on the patient's body regardless of his weight. Weight loss isn't recommended for a patient with a new or nonhealing wound; it's recommended only for a stable patient whose

Determining calorie needs

There are several different methods to determine a patient's caloric needs. Here are some calculations that can be used.

IDEAL BODY WEIGHT
Men—first 5 feet: 106 pounds
    each inch over 5 feet: add 6 pounds
Women—first 5 feet: 100 pounds
    each inch over 5 feet: add 5 pounds

ADJUSTED BODY WEIGHT
Men—(current weight – ideal body weight) $\times$ 0.38 + ideal body weight
Women—(current weight – ideal body weight) $\times$ 0.32 + ideal body weight

HARRIS-BENEDICT EQUATION
Basal metabolic rate (BMR)
Men—66.47 + (13.75 $\times$ weight in kg) + (5.0 $\times$ height in cm) – (6.76 $\times$ age)
Women—665.10 + (9.56 $\times$ weight in kg) + (1.85 $\times$ height in cm) – (4.68 $\times$ age)
Multiply the BMR by an activity factor and an injury factor to obtain the daily total requirements.
Activity factor—sedentary or bedridden patient: 1.2
    ambulatory patient: 1.3
Injury factor—recent surgery or trauma: 1.2 or 1.3
    wound or infection: 1.3 or 1.4
Note: If the patient has a body mass index (BMI) of 30 or higher, use adjusted body weight.

MIFFLIN-ST. JEOR EQUATION
Men—(10 $\times$ weight in kg) + (6.25 $\times$ height in cm) – (5 $\times$ age) + 5
Women—(10 $\times$ weight in kg) + (6.25 $\times$ height in cm) – (5 $\times$ age) – 161
Multiply with a combined activity/stress factor.

Determining calorie needs *(continued)*

Most hospital or bedridden patients: 1.2
Wound patients: 1.3 or 1.4
This equation is frequently used in intensive care patients.

CALORIES PER KILOGRAM
This equation is the quickest to use, and it can be used when the patient's height isn't available.
To maintain weight: 30 to 35 calories/kg
To gain weight: 35 to 40 calories/kg
To lose weight: 20 to 25 calories/kg
Note: If the patient's BMI is 30 or higher, use adjusted body weight.

---

wound is improving and whose albumin and prealbumin levels are within the normal range.

PROTEIN NEEDS

Protein is needed for repairing skin tissue and generating new skin cells for the healing process. White blood cells (WBCs) have a high protein level, which is why a patient's protein needs increase when a fever or infection develops. The patient will need protein that's higher than normal body requirements to initiate or continue the healing process. The body uses protein for repair and growth only after normal body functions are met.

Protein needs can also be determined by the severity of the wound. A patient with a partial-thickness wound requires less protein than a patient with a full-thickness wound.

Wounds with copious drainage can lose protein, so more protein is required. In addition, larger wounds require more protein to heal because of the greater surface area to replenish. Infection or an increase in the patient's

Complete and incomplete proteins

Complete proteins contain all essential amino acids. Incomplete proteins contain small amounts of essential amino acids, but they can be combined to make a complete protein.

COMPLETE PROTEIN SOURCES
Meat
Poultry
Fish
Eggs
Dairy
Soybeans
Legumes + seeds
Legumes + nuts
Legumes + dairy
Legumes + grains
Grains + dairy

INCOMPLETE PROTEIN SOURCES
Cereals and grains
Green, leafy vegetables
Legumes (beans)
Nuts
Fruits
Seeds

temperature or WBC count also requires a larger protein intake; use the upper end of the range in these cases.

Proteins are considered complete or incomplete. Complete proteins such as meats contain all the essential amino acids, whereas incomplete proteins such as legumes contain small amounts of one or more essential amino acids. Combinations of incomplete proteins such as a peanut butter and jelly sandwich, however, can provide all of the essential amino acids. Protein sources are important to consider when planning the patient's diet. (See *Complete and incomplete proteins.*)

FLUID NEEDS

Adequate fluid is required for maintaining proper skin turgor and for helping the body carry nutrients to the cells and eliminate wastes from the body. The average fluid need is 25 to 30 ml per kilogram of actual body weight. All cells require fluid to be effective, so fluid needs are always calculated according to the patient's actual weight, regardless of his BMI.

Some conditions require the patient to have a restricted fluid level to promote the healing process. Check with a practitioner before calculating fluid needs if the wound-care patient has pulmonary edema, heart failure, renal failure that requires hemodialysis, or pitting edema that's more than 1+.

3

WOUND ASSESSMENT AND MONITORING

Accurate wound assessment helps the health care team plan an appropriate care plan. It also guides the treatment of the wound and dictates the type of dressing used, how often the dressing is changed, and what drug (if any) needs to be used. The assessment is also important from a legal viewpoint. It conveys information to all caretakers about the state of the wound and allows the nurse to follow the improvement or worsening of the wound.

A wound assessment includes a total patient assessment, including lifestyle and other comorbid diagnoses. The cause of the wound should also be investigated and taken into consideration. This chapter tells you how to perform a wound assessment, including assessing healing potential, classifying the wound, assessing wound pain, recognizing complications, assessing successful healing, and documenting.

Assessing healing potential

Several factors influence the body's ability to heal itself, regardless of the type of injury suffered. You should include these elements in your wound assessment:
- immune status

- glucose levels, including glycosylated hemoglobin (HbA$_{1C}$)
- hydration
- nutrition
- blood albumin and prealbumin levels
- oxygen and vascular supply
- pain.

IMMUNE STATUS

The immune system plays a central role in wound healing. If the immune system is impaired due to such diseases as human immunodeficiency virus infection or as a result of chemotherapy or radiation, monitor the wound closely for impaired healing. Remember, chemotherapeutic drugs aren't only used to treat cancer, they're also used to treat inflammatory diseases such as rheumatoid arthritis. Corticosteroids may also depress immune system function.

GLUCOSE LEVELS

Glucose levels should be less than 180 mg/dl and HbA$_{1C}$ levels should be less than 7% for satisfactory healing, regardless of the cause of the wound. Levels of 180 mg/dl or more can impair the function of white blood cells (WBCs), which help prevent infection and are important in wound healing.

HYDRATION

Be sure to closely monitor and optimize the patient's hydration—successful healing depends on it. Skin and subcutaneous tissues need to be well hydrated from the inside. Dehydration impairs the healing process by slowing the body's metabolism; it also reduces skin turgor, leaving skin vulnerable to new wounds.

NUTRITION

Nutritional status helps you determine the patient's vulnerability to skin breakdown and the body's overall ability to heal. A comprehensive assessment of a patient's nutritional status is also helpful in planning effective care. For complete information on nutritional assessment, see chapter 2, Nutrition in wound care.

Nutrition is complex. If your assessment indicates that the patient's nutritional status places him at risk for skin damage or for delayed wound healing, collaborate with a dietitian to develop the best possible treatment plan.

ALBUMIN LEVELS

Albumin and prealbumin levels are essential factors in wound assessment for two important reasons:

■ First, skin is primarily constructed of protein, and albumin is a protein. If albumin levels are low, the body lacks an important building block for skin repair.

■ Second, albumin is the blood component that provides colloid osmotic pressure—the force that prevents fluid from leaking out of blood vessels into nearby tissues. (See *A closer look at albumin*.)

If albumin levels fall below 3.5 g/dl, edema may occur, which compromises wound healing. As fluid leaks out of the bloodstream into tissues, the patient is also at risk for developing hypotension. If blood pressure falls to the point where adequate blood flow is no longer maintained through the capillaries near the wound, healing slows or stops.

OXYGEN AND VASCULAR SUPPLY

Healing requires oxygen—it's that simple. Therefore, anything that impedes full oxygenation also impedes healing. Assessment should consider any factor that can reduce the

A closer look at albumin

Albumin, a large protein molecule, acts like a magnet to attract water and hold it inside the blood vessel.

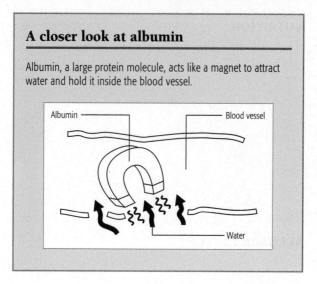

amount of oxygen available for healing; examples of possible problems include:

- impaired gas exchange, causing decreased oxygen levels in the blood
- hemoglobin levels too low to transport adequate oxygen
- low blood pressure that fails to drive oxygenated blood through capillaries
- insufficient arterial and capillary supply in the area of the wound.

Any one or a combination of these problems can deprive the wound of the oxygen needed for successful healing.

Smoking is a modifiable factor that impedes oxygenation of the wound. Explain to a patient who smokes these ways in which smoking affects wound healing:

- ▣ Nicotine is a powerful vasoconstrictor that narrows peripheral blood vessels, thereby compromising blood flow to the skin.
- ▣ Because hemoglobin binds more easily to the carbon monoxide in cigarette smoke than to oxygen, the blood carries far less oxygen than it should.
- ▣ Lung tissue damaged by smoke doesn't function optimally, resulting in decreased oxygenation.

PAIN

To promote patient comfort, control your patient's pain as effectively as possible. Pain control also has a practical purpose. In response to pain, the body releases epinephrine, a powerful vasoconstrictor. Vasoconstriction reduces blood flow to the wound. When pain is relieved, vasoconstriction subsides, blood vessels dilate, and blood flow to the wound improves.

Classifying wounds

The words you choose to describe observations of a specific wound have to communicate the same thing to other health care team members, insurance companies, regulators, the patient's family and, ultimately, the patient himself. This is difficult when even wound care experts debate the descriptive phrases they use: "slough" or "eschar"? "Undermining" or "tunneling"? How much drainage is "moderate"? Is the color green or yellow?

Wounds can best be classified by using the basic system described here, which focuses on three fundamental characteristics:

- ▣ cause
- ▣ age
- ▣ depth.

CAUSE

The two basic causes of wounds are surgical and nonsurgical. Surgical wounds usually heal more quickly than nonsurgical wounds. Both types of wounds require careful monitoring to prevent complications.

AGE

When determining the age of a wound, first confirm whether it's acute or chronic. This can become problematic, however, if the assessment is based only on time: when does an acute wound becomes a chronic wound?

A wound is considered to be acute if it's new or making progress as expected; a chronic wound is one that isn't healing in a timely manner. In a chronic wound, healing has slowed or stopped and the wound isn't getting smaller and shallower. Even if the wound bed appears healthy, red, and moist, if healing fails to progress, it's a chronic wound.

Chronic wounds don't heal as easily as acute wounds. The drainage in chronic wounds contains a greater amount of destructive enzymes, and fibroblasts—the cells that act as the architects in wound healing—seem to lose their effectiveness. The fibroblasts are less effective at producing collagen, divide less often, and send fewer signals to other cells instructing them to divide and fill the wound. Thus, the wound changes from one that's vigorous and ready to heal to one that's lazy.

DEPTH

Wound depth is another fundamental characteristic used to classify wounds. Record wound depth as partial- or full-thickness. (See *Classifying wound depth*, page 54.)

Wound depth also allows pressure ulcers to be staged according to the classification system developed by the National Pressure Ulcer Advisory Panel, or NPUAP.

EXPERT TIPS

Classifying wound depth

Wounds are classified as partial-thickness or full-thickness based on the depth of the wound. Partial-thickness wounds involve only the epidermis or extend into the dermis but not through it. Full-thickness wounds extend through the dermis into tissues beneath and may expose adipose tissue, muscle, or bone. These diagrams illustrate the relative depth of both classifications.

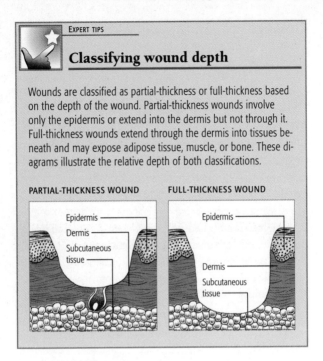

PARTIAL-THICKNESS WOUND

Epidermis
Dermis
Subcutaneous tissue

FULL-THICKNESS WOUND

Epidermis

Dermis
Subcutaneous tissue

Partial-thickness wounds

Partial-thickness wounds normally heal quickly because they involve only the epidermal layer of the skin or extend through the epidermis into (but not through) the dermis. The dermis remains at least partially intact to generate the new epidermis needed to close the wound. Partial-thickness wounds are also less susceptible to infection because part of the body's first level of defense (the skin) is still intact. These wounds tend to be painful, however, and need protection from the air to reduce pain.

Full-thickness wounds

Full-thickness wounds penetrate completely through the skin into underlying tissues. The wound may expose adipose tissue (fat), muscle, tendon, or bone. In the abdomen, adipose tissue or omentum (the covering of the bowel) may be visible. If the omentum is penetrated, the bowel may protrude through the wound (evisceration). Granulation tissue may be visible if the wound has started to heal.

Full-thickness wounds heal by granulation and contraction, which require more body resources and more time than the healing of partial-thickness wounds. When assessing a full-thickness wound, report the depth as well as the length and width of the wound.

Assessing wounds

Gathering information about a wound requires use of almost every one of your five senses. Assess the wound bed, drainage, and patient's pain. Assess the wound bed and surrounding skin only after they've been cleaned.

In the course of a wound assessment, you gather much useful information about the patient, his environment, the characteristics of his wound, and his current status in the healing process. Your assessment has created a picture of the wound that accurately depicts your patient and his current status. Consistently record all observations. (See *Documenting wounds,* page 56.)

In assessing the wound bed, record information about:

■ wound length, width, and depth
■ tunneling and undermining
■ appearance
■ wound drainage
■ odor
■ margins and surrounding skin.

Documenting wounds

Use this mnemonic device, WOUND PICTURE, to help you recall and organize all of the key facts that should be included in your documentation.

- *W*ound or ulcer location
- *O*dor? (in room or just when wound is uncovered)
- *U*lcer category, stage (for pressure ulcer) or classification (for diabetic ulcer), and depth (partial-thickness or full-thickness)
- *N*ecrotic tissue?
- *D*imension of wound (shape, length, width, depth); drainage color, consistency, and amount (scant, moderate, large)
- *P*ain? (when it occurs, what relieves it, patient's description, patient's rating on scale of 0 to 10)
- *I*nduration? (surrounding tissue hard or soft)
- *C*olor of wound bed (red, yellow, black, or combination)
- *T*unneling? (record length and direction—toward patient's right, left, head, feet)
- *U*ndermining? (record length and direction, using clock references to describe)
- *R*edness or other discoloration in surrounding skin?
- *E*dge of skin loose or tightly adhered? Edges flat or rolled under?

Length, width, and depth

Because accurately recording wound dimensions is important, many health care facilities use photography as a tool in wound assessment. If photography is available in your facility, include it in your assessment of wound characteristics. Some photographic techniques produce a picture with a grid overlay that's useful for measuring. However, there are qualities of the wound that can't be recorded by a camera. (See *Photography in wound assessment.*)

Wounds are commonly measured with a tape measure. Make sure it's a disposable device to prevent contamination and cross-contamination. Record the length of the

EXPERT TIPS

Photography in wound assessment

If photographing wounds is a routine part of your wound documentation system, remember that your assessment skills and personal observations are still essential. Many wound characteristics can't be recorded accurately—or at all—on film. These include:

- location
- depth
- tunnel measurement
- odor
- feel of surrounding tissue
- pain.

All of this information is needed for the health care team to make sound treatment decisions.

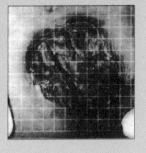

wound as the longest overall distance across the wound (regardless of orientation), and record the width as the longest measurement perpendicular (at a right angle) to the length measurement. (See *Measuring a wound,* page 58.)

Record observed areas of discoloration of the intact skin around the wound opening separately—not as part of the wound bed. Record all measurements in centimeters.

Another way to measure the wound is to use wound tracing (wound margins are traced on a sheet of clear plastic). Use the tracing to calculate an approximate wound area. Although this method provides a rough estimate only, it's simple and fairly quick.

To measure the depth of the wound, gently insert a sterile cotton-tipped swab into the deepest portion of the wound and then carefully mark the stick where it meets

Measuring a wound

When measuring a wound, first determine the longest distance across the open area of the wound—regardless of orientation. Note the line used to illustrate this length in the photograph.

A wound's width is simply the longest distance across the wound at a right angle to the length. Note the relationship of length and width in the photograph. Also note the area of reddened, intact skin and white macerated skin. These areas would be measured and recorded as surrounding erythema and maceration—not as part of the wound itself. In this full-thickness ischial pressure ulcer, also record a depth and note areas of tunneling or undermining.

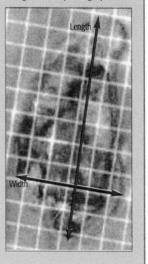

the edge of the skin. Remove the swab and measure the distance from the mark to the end to determine depth.

Tunneling and undermining

Tunnels, or sinus tracts (extensions of the wound bed into adjacent tissue), and undermining (areas of the wound bed that extend under the skin) are measured like wound depth. Carefully insert a sterile cotton-tipped swab to the bottom of the tunnel or to the end of the undermined area; mark the stick, and measure the distance from the mark to the end of the swab. If a tunnel is large, palpate it with a gloved finger rather than a swab because the end of the tunnel can be better felt with a finger. This also avoids damaging the tissue.

Appearance

Identify tissue present in the wound bed in percentages and identify structures in the wound bed. Avascular and necrotic tissue, both of which are nonviable, are seen in two colors: yellow and gray. Fibrin slough is stringy tissue that adheres to the wound bed and may be yellow, tan, gray, or black. Eschar is black, hardened tissue in the wound bed. Vascular tissue shows signs of granulation and is generally pink or red. (See *Tailoring wound care to your wound assessment*, page 60.)

The texture of the wound bed provides as much information about the wound and healing as its color. If smooth red tissue is noted in a partial-thickness wound, it's most likely the dermis. In a full-thickness wound, it's probably muscle tissue, not granulation tissue. In a full-thickness wound, healthy granulation tissue has a soft, bumpy appearance like the surface of a bowl of tapioca, only red and is a sign of proper healing.

During each assessment, focus on the cause of the wound to ensure that all factors that can influence healing have been considered. For example, if you're assessing a patient with a venous insufficiency ulcer, measure the wound and the calf circumference regularly to determine whether efforts to reduce edema are succeeding. The best interventions for a venous insufficiency ulcer won't heal the wound if edema is left unchecked.

Similarly, if you're assessing the wound of a patient with diabetes, ensure that his glucose level is well controlled and that the calluses that tend to build up around diabetic foot ulcers are removed regularly. Otherwise, healing will be impeded.

Tailoring wound care to your wound assessment

With any wound, you can promote healing by keeping the wound moist, clean, and free of debris. For open wounds, identifying the condition of the wound bed can guide the specific management approach to aid healing. Consider the amount of drainage when selecting therapies.

WOUND BED CONDITION	MANAGEMENT TECHNIQUE
Pink or red	• Cover the wound to keep it clean and protected. Keep the wound moist. • For minimal drainage, use a transparent film, hydrocolloid, or hydrogel dressing. • Foams, alginates, and hydrofibers absorb drainage. • Remember, beefy red may indicate bioburden of the wound bed and a topical antimicrobial may be warranted.
Fibrin slough	• Debride wound using enzymatic debridement or pulsatile lavage. • Use a moisture-retentive dressing to stimulate autolytic debridement. • Use an alginate or hydrofiber to absorb drainage and support autolytic debridement. • Topical antimicrobials may also be indicated in this wound.
Eschar	• Depending on location, eschar needs to be debrided by conservative sharp, enzymatic, or pulsatile lavage methods. • For wounds with inadequate blood supply and noninfected heel ulcers, keep clean and dry. • Topical antimicrobials may also be indicated in this wound as the tissue begins to break down.

In other words, "don't miss the forest for the trees." When focusing on specific wound characteristics, describing them, and tracking the healing process, don't lose sight of the patient's overall condition.

Other causes of wounds include allergies, autoimmune disorders, and infectious processes. The patient is usually the best source of information about the cause of the wound. If he doesn't know or remember, ask him about new drugs he's taking, skin creams, animal bites, or scrapes or punctures. The family may also be able to provide information regarding a wound if the patient is confused or has an altered level of consciousness.

Drainage

The wound bed should be moist—but not overly moist. Moisture allows the cells and chemicals needed for healing to move about the wound surface.

In dry wound beds, cells involved in healing, which normally exist in a fluid environment, can't move. WBCs can't fight infection, enzymes such as collagenase can't break down dead material, and macrophages can't carry away debris. The wound edges curl up to preserve moisture remaining in the edge and epithelial cells (new skin cells) fail to grow over and cover the wound. Healing stops and necrotic tissue builds up.

Excess moisture poses a different problem. It floods the wound and spills out onto the skin, where the constant moisture causes the death of skin cells.

Consider the texture of the drainage as well. If the drainage has a thick, creamy texture, the wound contains an excessive amount of bacteria; however, this doesn't necessarily mean a clinically significant infection exists. Document the characteristics of the drainage. It might be creamy because it contains WBCs that have killed bacteria. The drainage is also contaminated with surface bacteria that naturally live in moist environments on the human body. Because of this bacterial colonization, guidelines developed by the Agency for Health Care Policy and Research, now the Agency for Healthcare Research and Quality, rec-

---

EXPERT TIPS

Drainage descriptors

This chart provides terminology that you can use to describe the color and consistency of wound drainage.

DESCRIPTION	COLOR AND CONSISTENCY
Serous	● Clear or light yellow ● Thin and watery
Sanguineous	● Red (with fresh blood) ● Thin
Serosanguineous	● Pink to light red ● Thin ● Watery
Purulent	● Creamy yellow, green, white, or tan ● Thick and opaque

---

ommend against using swab cultures to identify wound infections. Nonetheless, some practitioners still order swab cultures because they're inexpensive and easy to collect.

Ideally, obtain a swab of the clear fluid expressed from the wound tissue after it has been thoroughly cleaned. This is more likely to produce a sample of the bacteria in question. Punch biopsy of tissue or needle aspiration of fluid may also be used. These methods require more skill but are more likely to reveal accurate results.

To begin collecting information about wound drainage, inspect the dressing as it's removed and record answers to such questions as:

■ Is the drainage well contained, or is it oozing from the edges? If it's oozing, consider using a more absorbent dressing.

■ If an occlusive dressing was used, were the dressing
  edges well sealed? (A hydrocolloid in the gluteal cleft
  area becomes a greenhouse for bacteria if the edges are
  loose.) If the patient has fecal incontinence, it's even
  more important to note the seal status.
■ Is the dressing saturated or dry?
■ How much drainage is there: a scant, moderate, or
  large amount?
■ What are the color and consistency of the drainage?
  (See *Drainage descriptors.*)

Odor

If kept clean, a noninfected wound usually produces little,
if any, odor. (One exception is the odor normally present
under a hydrocolloid dressing that develops as a by-product
of the degradation process.) A newly detected odor might
be a sign of infection; record it and report it to the primary
nurse and the practitioner. When documenting wound
odor, it's important to include when the odor was noted
and whether it went away with wound cleaning.

   If an odor develops, it can present an embarrassing or
otherwise uncomfortable situation for the patient as well
as his family, guests, and roommate. If an odor is noticed,
or if the patient notices one, use an odor eliminator. Odor
eliminators differ from air fresheners in that they aren't
scents that mask odors but rather compounds that bind
with, and neutralize, the molecules responsible for the
odor.

Margins and surrounding skin

When assessing wound margins, look for skin that's
smooth—not rolled—and tightly adherent to the wound
bed. Rolled skin may indicate that the wound bed is too
dry. Loose skin at the edges may indicate additional shearing injury (separation of skin layers), possibly due to a

rough transfer or repositioning. In this case, improve transfer and repositioning techniques to prevent recurrence.

The skin color around the wound can signal impending problems that can impede healing:

▪ White skin indicates maceration, or too much moisture, and signals the need for a protective barrier around the wound and a more absorbent dressing.

▪ Red skin can indicate inflammation, injury (for example, tape burn, excessive pressure, or chemical exposure), or infection. Inflammation is healthy only during the inflammatory phase of healing—not after.

▪ Purple skin can indicate bruising, one sign of trauma.

During an assessment of the area around the wound, the fingers can pick up valuable information. For example, with a gloved finger, gently probe the tissue around the wound bed to determine if it's soft or hard (indurated). Indurated tissue, even in the absence of erythema (redness), is an indication of infection. Similarly, if the patient has dark skin, it may be impossible to see color cues. Probe the area around the wound bed and compare the feel with surrounding healthy skin. A tender area of skin that appears shiny and feels hard may indicate inflammation in a dark-skinned patient.

Assessing wound pain

Assessing patient pain is an important part of wound assessment. Note the pain associated with the injury and also that associated with healing and with therapies used to promote healing. To fully understand your patient's pain, ask him about his pain. Then, watch to see how he responds to pain and the therapies provided. Record your findings. (See *How to assess pain.*)

How to assess pain

To properly assess patient pain, consider the patient's descriptions and your own observations of his reaction to pain and treatments.

TALK TO YOUR PATIENT
Begin your pain assessment by asking your patient these questions:
● Where's the pain located? How long does it last? How often does it occur?
● What does the pain feel like? (Let the patient describe it; don't prompt.)
● What relieves the pain? What makes it worse?
● How do you usually get relief?
● How would you rate your pain on a scale of 0 to 10, with 0 representing no pain and 10 representing the worst pain?

Talking with the patient about his pain in this manner helps him define his pain, for himself as well as you, and helps you evaluate the effectiveness of therapies used to relieve pain.

MONITOR AND OBSERVE YOUR PATIENT
As you work with the patient, observe his responses to pain and to interventions intended to relieve pain.

Behavioral responses to watch for include:
● altered body position
● moaning
● sighing
● grimacing
● withdrawing from painful stimuli
● crying
● restlessness
● muscle twitching
● immobility.

Sympathetic responses, normally associated with mild to moderate pain, include:
● pallor
● elevated blood pressure
● dilated pupils
● tension in skeletal muscles
● dyspnea (shortness of breath)
● tachycardia (rapid heart beat)
● diaphoresis (sweating).

Parasympathetic responses, which are more common in cases of severe, deep pain, include:
● pallor
● lower than normal blood pressure
● bradycardia (slower than normal heartbeat)
● nausea and vomiting
● weakness
● dizziness
● loss of consciousness.

If your patient is conscious and can communicate, have him rate his pain before and during each dressing change. If his pain level is higher before the dressing change, it may indicate an impending infection, even before other signs appear.

If your patient says the dressing change itself is painful, the patient should receive drugs before the procedure or the dressing technique should be changed. Document the patient's pain and report it to the primary nurse and practitioner. Less painful methods of removing dead tissue exist but, if the patient's pain isn't documented and communicated, wet-to-dry debridement orders may stand and the patient may suffer unnecessary discomfort.

When removing adherent dressings, it's less painful when the dressing is soaked or, over intact skin, an adhesive remover is used. Keep the skin taut. Press down on the skin to release the dressing, rather than pull the dressing off. If the patient still says that dressing removal is painful, the team may wish to choose a less adherent type of dressing.

Recognizing complications

It's important to monitor wound status to identify signs and symptoms of complications or failure to heal as early as possible. Early intervention improves the likelihood of resolving complications successfully and getting the healing process back on track.

You'll conduct your reassessments using the same criteria used in the initial assessment, with an added advantage—perspective. Careful monitoring can help you catch failure to heal early so you can intervene appropriately. (See *Recognizing failure to heal.*)

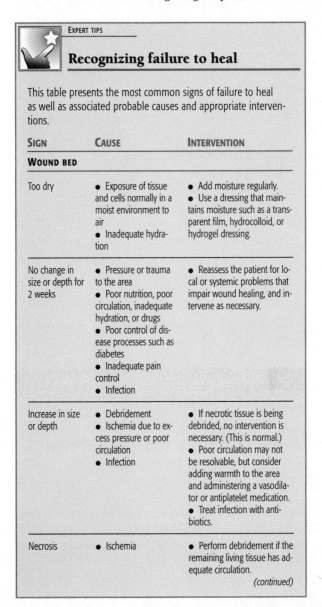

EXPERT TIPS

Recognizing failure to heal

This table presents the most common signs of failure to heal as well as associated probable causes and appropriate interventions.

SIGN	CAUSE	INTERVENTION
WOUND BED		
Too dry	● Exposure of tissue and cells normally in a moist environment to air ● Inadequate hydration	● Add moisture regularly. ● Use a dressing that maintains moisture such as a transparent film, hydrocolloid, or hydrogel dressing.
No change in size or depth for 2 weeks	● Pressure or trauma to the area ● Poor nutrition, poor circulation, inadequate hydration, or drugs ● Poor control of disease processes such as diabetes ● Inadequate pain control ● Infection	● Reassess the patient for local or systemic problems that impair wound healing, and intervene as necessary.
Increase in size or depth	● Debridement ● Ischemia due to excess pressure or poor circulation ● Infection	● If necrotic tissue is being debrided, no intervention is necessary. (This is normal.) ● Poor circulation may not be resolvable, but consider adding warmth to the area and administering a vasodilator or antiplatelet medication. ● Treat infection with antibiotics.
Necrosis	● Ischemia	● Perform debridement if the remaining living tissue has adequate circulation.

(continued)

Recognizing failure to heal (*continued*)

SIGN	CAUSE	INTERVENTION
WOUND BED (*continued*)		
Increase in drainage or change of drainage color from clear to purulent	• Autolytic or enzymatic debridement • Infection	• No intervention is necessary if caused by autolytic or enzymatic debridement. Increase in drainage or change of drainage color is expected because of the breakdown of dead tissue. • If debridement isn't the cause, assess the wound for infection.
Tunneling	• Pressure over bony prominences • Presence of foreign body • Deep infection	• Protect the area from pressure. • Irrigate and inspect the tunnel as carefully as possible for a hidden suture or leftover bit of dressing material. • If the tunnel doesn't shorten in length each week, thoroughly clean and obtain a tissue biopsy for infection and, with a chronic wound, for possible malignancy.
WOUND EDGES		
Red, hot skin; tenderness; induration	• Inflammation due to excess pressure or infection	• If pressure relief doesn't resolve the inflammation within 24 hours, topical antimicrobial therapy may be indicated.
White skin (maceration)	• Excess moisture	• Protect the skin with petrolatum ointment or barrier wipe. • If practical, obtain an order for a more absorptive dressing.

Recognizing failure to heal (*continued*)

SIGN	CAUSE	INTERVENTION
WOUND EDGES (*continued*)		
Rolled skin edges	● Too-dry wound bed	● Obtain an order for moisture-retentive dressings. ● If rolling isn't resolved in 1 week, debridement of the edges may be necessary.
Undermining or ecchymosis of surrounding skin (loose or bruised skin edges)	● Excess shearing force to the area	● Protect the area, especially during patient transfers.

Success or failure of the healing process has a tremendous impact on the patient's quality of life as well as his family's quality of life. Early intervention can mean that a patient with a diabetic foot ulcer can avoid amputation or a paraplegic patient with an ischial ulcer can once again sit up and lead an active life.

Chronic ulcers pose a particularly difficult problem, not only for individual practitioners but also for the health care industry. Treating chronic ulcers is expensive because they're difficult or impossible to heal. Consequently, the people paying the largest portion of the bill—the government and insurance companies—are placing increased emphasis on early intervention and prevention.

Recognizing successful healing

Now that you know what to look for when things aren't going well, let's take a look at what you can expect to see when healing is progressing smoothly. In this case, your patient:

■ is well hydrated, well nourished, comfortable, and warm

■ is well managed for associated or contributing diseases, such as diabetes, heart failure, or renal failure

■ exhibits normal immune system response.

In addition, the wound itself:

■ receives the oxygen and nutrients it needs (adequate vascular supply)

■ is moist and protected from the environment

■ is free from necrotic tissue.

These conditions optimize wound healing. By using the assessment techniques presented in this chapter, you'll be a part of this success.

Wound healing isn't a simple matter to coordinate. Through vigilance and consistent assessment and documentation, success is much more likely. By using most of your senses, you can have a tremendous influence on whether a wound heals or becomes chronic and harder to manage. Recognizing red flags that warn of failure to heal, and knowing the appropriate interventions, make you a part of the winning wound healing team.

MONITORING HEALING

The next step is to monitor the patient throughout the healing process, periodically reassessing his status and documenting progress to full healing. Not only is this an excellent way to determine progress and the usefulness of interventions, but it's also a requirement for some regulatory agencies such as the Centers for Medicare and Medicaid Services (CMS).

Your initial assessment sets the benchmark for subsequent monitoring and reassessment activities. One assessment is a static report. A series of assessments, however, becomes a moving picture illustrating the dynamic aspect of the healing process. In this way, all members of the health care team can see progress toward healing (or failure to heal), developing complications, and the relative success of interventions. The view will depend on the accuracy, quality, and consistency of your documentation.

The prospect of monitoring, reassessing, and documenting over time may seem exciting or daunting, depending on your energy level. But take heart, several good research-based documentation tools are available—or your facility may have its own—to help you manage the task.

Documenting wounds

Most wound documentation tools used in the United States focus on pressure ulcers. Pressure ulcers were selected as the basis because of the tremendous impact they've had on countless patients' lives and the health care system. Pressure ulcers are painful, typically chronic, life-disrupting, and expensive to treat—both in dollars and in amount of time spent by providers. They're also usually preventable.

Pressure Ulcer Scale for Healing

The Pressure Ulcer Scale for Healing (PUSH) tool was developed and revised by NPUAP and is only applicable to pressure ulcers. (See *PUSH tool*, pages 72 and 73.)

When working with this tool, you develop three scores: one for the surface area (length × width), one for the drainage amount, and one for the tissue type in the wound during each review. The sum of these scores yields a total score for the wound on a given day. This score is then plotted on a pressure ulcer healing record and heal-

PUSH tool

The beauty of the Pressure Ulcer Scale for Healing (PUSH) tool is its simplicity. It's quick and easy to score.

Patient
name _David Quinn_

User
location _Sunview Nursing Home_

Patient I.D. _0162386_

Date _1/3/07_

DIRECTIONS

Observe and measure the pressure ulcer. Categorize the ulcer with respect to surface area, exudate, and type of wound tissue. Record a subscore for each of the ulcer characteristics. Add the subscores to obtain the total score. A comparison of total scores measured over time provides an indication of the improvement or deterioration in pressure ulcer healing.

Length × width	**0** 0 cm²	**1** <0.3 cm²	**2** 0.3 to 0.6 cm²	**3** 0.7 to 1.0 cm²	**4** 1.1 to 2.0 cm²	**5** 2.1 to 3.0 cm²	Subscore 3
		6 3.1 to 4.0 cm²	**7** 4.1 to 8.0 cm²	**8** 8.1 to 12.0 cm²	**9** 12.1 to 24.0 cm²	**10** >24.0 cm²	
Exudate amount	**0** None	**1** Light	**2** Moderate	**3** Heavy			Subscore 2
Tissue type	**0** Closed	**1** Epithelial tissue	**2** Granulation tissue	**3** Slough	**4** Necrotic tissue		Subscore 1
							Total score: 6

LENGTH × WIDTH

Measure the greatest length (head-to-toe) and the greatest width (side-to-side) using a centimeter ruler. Multiply these two measurements (length × width) to obtain an estimate of surface area in square centimeters (cm²). Don't guess! Always use a

PUSH tool *(continued)*

centimeter ruler and always use the same method each time the ulcer is measured.

EXUDATE AMOUNT

Estimate the amount of exudate (drainage) present after removal of the dressing and before applying any topical agent to the ulcer. Estimate the exudate as *none, light, moderate,* or *heavy*.

TISSUE TYPE

This refers to the types of tissue that are present in the wound (ulcer) bed. Score as a 4 if necrotic tissue is present. Score as a 3 if slough is present and necrotic tissue is absent. Score as a 2 if the wound is clean and contains granulation tissue. Score a superficial wound that's re-epithelializing as a 1. When the wound is closed, score it as a 0.

4–Necrotic tissue (eschar): Black, brown, or tan tissue that adheres firmly to the wound bed or ulcer edges and may be either firmer or softer than surrounding tissue

3–Slough: Yellow or white tissue that adheres to the ulcer bed in strings or thick clumps or is mucinous

2–Granulation tissue: Pink or beefy red tissue with a shiny, moist, granular appearance

1–Epithelial tissue: For superficial ulcers, new pink or shiny tissue (skin) that grows in from the edges or as islands on the ulcer surface

0–Closed or resurfaced: Completely covered wound with epithelium (new skin)

Adapted with permission from PUSH tool version 3.0, © 1998 National Pressure Ulcer Advisory Panel, Reston, Va.

ing graph. By recording and reviewing scores over time, you can determine the pace of progress toward healing.

NPUAP is working with CMS to incorporate the PUSH tool in Resident Assessment Protocols to accompany the Minimum Data Set used in long-term care facilities.

Pressure Sore Status Tool

The Pressure Sore Status Tool (PSST) allows you to track scores for 11 factors over time. These factors are each scored based on a number scale, and the scores are added. The total score reflects overall wound status.

The PSST is a precise record of wound changes and is fairly time consuming to complete. Consequently, it's used more in research than in clinical practice.

Wound Healing Scale

The Wound Healing Scale is a simple classification system that combines a designation for wound stage, or thickness, with a tissue descriptor. For example, a stage 3 pressure ulcer containing necrotic tissue is recorded as 3N. Using this tool, you can track the general direction of healing by noting, for example, that this week the wound is an FG (full-thickness with granulation tissue), whereas last week it was an FN (full-thickness with necrotic tissue). Although the tool was developed initially for use with pressure ulcers, it includes modifiers that allow it to be used for all types of wounds.

Sussman Wound Healing Tool

The Sussman Wound Healing Tool was developed to help physical therapists track pressure ulcer healing. This tool lists 10 wound attributes and classifies each as "good" or "not good" in terms of wound healing. For example, granulation tissue is classified "good" and undermining is classified "not good." During each assessment, record your findings for each of the 10 attributes that apply to the patient; over time, this provides a picture of healing or failure to heal.

4

BASIC WOUND CARE PROCEDURES

Wound care orders are typically written by physicians, podiatrists, nurse practitioners, and physician assistants. However, policies and procedures related to skin and wound care activities are commonly written by registered nurses and performed by registered and licensed practical nurses. The practitioner in charge reviews and approves these policies and procedures. Many facilities now have specific policies and procedures for different types of wounds.

When you're presented with an order to provide wound care, it should include this essential information:

- wound description, including cause, location, appearance, and size
- cleaning solution and method
- type of dressing for the primary and, if needed, secondary layers
- topical drugs needed
- frequency of dressing changes
- time frame for evaluating and changing dressings.

Typically, if the wound hasn't changed in 2 weeks, the patient's condition and wound should be reassessed and the management plan should be revised accordingly. New orders may be needed. If no healing progress is apparent after 4 to 12 weeks of treatment, referral to a wound-care specialist is recommended.

Determining a wound-care plan

Wound care is an art and a science. It's based on the whole patient: his condition, his needs, and the wound profile. The goals of wound care include:

- promoting wound healing by controlling or eliminating causative factors
- preventing or managing infection
- removing nonviable tissue (debridement) as needed
- enhancing adequate blood supply
- providing nutritional and fluid support
- establishing and maintaining a clean, moist, protected wound bed
- managing wound fluid or drainage
- maintaining the skin surrounding the wound to ensure it remains dry and intact.

With any wound, healing may be promoted by keeping the wound moist, clean, and free from debris. However, requirements for providing wound care vary according to the patient assessment and the nature of the wound. (See *Guide to making wound care decisions.*)

Basic wound care

Basic wound care centers on cleaning and dressing the wound. Because open wounds are contaminated with bacteria, observe clean technique using clean, nonsterile gloves during wound care unless sterile dressing changes are specified. Always follow standard precautions.

The goal of wound cleaning is to remove debris and contaminants from the wound without damaging healthy

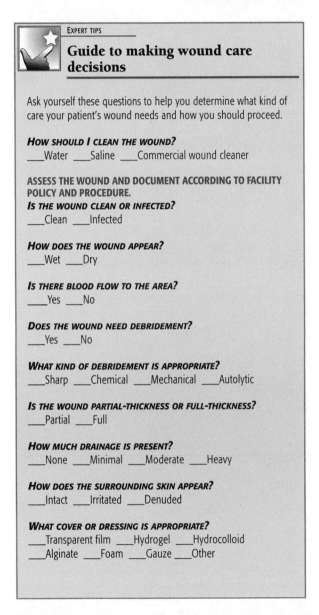

EXPERT TIPS

Guide to making wound care decisions

Ask yourself these questions to help you determine what kind of care your patient's wound needs and how you should proceed.

HOW SHOULD I CLEAN THE WOUND?
___Water ___Saline ___Commercial wound cleaner

ASSESS THE WOUND AND DOCUMENT ACCORDING TO FACILITY POLICY AND PROCEDURE.
IS THE WOUND CLEAN OR INFECTED?
___Clean ___Infected

HOW DOES THE WOUND APPEAR?
___Wet ___Dry

IS THERE BLOOD FLOW TO THE AREA?
___Yes ___No

DOES THE WOUND NEED DEBRIDEMENT?
___Yes ___No

WHAT KIND OF DEBRIDEMENT IS APPROPRIATE?
___Sharp ___Chemical ___Mechanical ___Autolytic

IS THE WOUND PARTIAL-THICKNESS OR FULL-THICKNESS?
___Partial ___Full

HOW MUCH DRAINAGE IS PRESENT?
___None ___Minimal ___Moderate ___Heavy

HOW DOES THE SURROUNDING SKIN APPEAR?
___Intact ___Irritated ___Denuded

WHAT COVER OR DRESSING IS APPROPRIATE?
___Transparent film ___Hydrogel ___Hydrocolloid
___Alginate ___Foam ___Gauze ___Other

tissue. The wound should be cleaned initially; repeat cleaning as needed or before a new dressing is applied.

The basic purpose of a dressing is to provide the best environment for the body to heal itself. This environment should be considered before a dressing is selected. Functions of a wound dressing include:

- protecting the wound from contamination and trauma
- providing compression if bleeding or swelling is anticipated
- applying medications
- absorbing drainage or debrided necrotic tissue
- filling or packing the wound
- protecting the skin surrounding the wound.

The cardinal rule is to keep wound tissue moist and surrounding tissue dry. Ideally, a dressing should keep the wound moist, absorb drainage or debris, conform to the wound, and be adhesive to surrounding skin yet also be easily removable. It should also be user-friendly, require minimal changes, decrease the need for a secondary dressing layer, and be cost-effective and comfortable for the patient.

EQUIPMENT

- Hypoallergenic tape or elastic netting
- Overbed table
- Piston-type irrigating system
- Two pairs of gloves
- Cleaning solution (such as normal saline solution) as ordered
- Sterile 4″ × 4″ gauze pads
- Selected topical dressing
- Linen-saver pads
- Impervious plastic trash bag
- Disposable wound-measuring device

PREPARATION

Assemble the equipment at the patient's bedside. Use clean or sterile technique, depending on facility policy and wound care orders. Cut tape into strips for securing dressings. Loosen lids on cleaning solutions and medications for easy removal. Attach an impervious plastic trash bag to the overbed table to hold used dressings and refuse.

IMPLEMENTATION

■ Before a dressing change, wash your hands and review the principles of standard precautions.

Cleaning the wound

■ Clean wounds with each dressing change; however, skin grafts should be changed only when ordered by the surgeon.

■ Provide privacy, and explain the procedure to the patient to allay his fears and promote cooperation.

■ Position the patient to maximize his comfort while allowing easy access to the wound site.

■ Cover bed linens with a linen-saver pad to prevent soiling.

■ Open the cleaning solution container and carefully pour cleaning solution into a bowl to avoid splashing. The bowl may be clean or sterile, depending on facility policy. (See *Choosing a cleaning solution,* page 80.)

■ Open the packages of supplies.

■ Put on gloves.

■ Gently roll or lift an edge of the soiled dressing to obtain a starting point. Support adjacent skin while gently releasing the soiled dressing from the skin. When possible, remove the dressing in the direction of hair growth.

Choosing a cleaning solution

The most commonly used cleaning agent is sterile normal saline solution, which provides a moist environment, promotes granulation tissue formation, and causes minimal fluid shifts in healthy adults.

Antiseptic solutions may damage tissue and delay healing but are sometimes used for cleaning infected or newly contaminated wounds. Examples of antiseptic solutions include:

● *hydrogen peroxide* (commonly used half-strength), which irrigates the wound and aids in mechanical debridement (its foaming action also warms the wound, promoting vasodilation and reducing inflammation)

● *acetic acid,* which treats *Pseudomonas* infection

● *sodium hypochlorite* (Dakin's fluid), an antiseptic that also slightly dissolves necrotic tissue (this unstable solution must be freshly prepared every 24 hours)

● *povidone-iodine,* a broad-spectrum, fast-acting antimicrobial (watch for patient sensitivity to this solution; also, protect the surrounding skin from contact because this solution can dry and stain the skin).

■ Discard the soiled dressing and your contaminated gloves in the impervious plastic trash bag to avoid contaminating the clean or sterile field.

■ Put on a clean pair of gloves (sterile or nonsterile, depending on facility policy or the wound care order).

■ Inspect the wound. Note the color, amount, and odor of drainage and necrotic debris.

■ Inspect the skin around the wound. Note redness, heat, moisture, irritation, or damage from the dressing.

■ Fold a sterile 4″ × 4″ gauze pad into quarters and grasp it with your fingers. Make sure the folded edge faces outward.

- Dip the folded gauze into the cleaning solution. Alternatively, use a wound cleaning solution in a spray bottle or a piston-type syringe.
- When cleaning, be sure to move from the least-contaminated area to the most-contaminated area. For a linear-shaped wound, such as an incision, gently wipe from top to bottom in one motion, starting directly over the wound and moving outward. For an open wound, such as a pressure ulcer, gently wipe in concentric circles, again starting directly over the wound and moving outward.
- Discard the gauze pad in the plastic trash bag.
- Using a clean gauze pad for each wiping motion, repeat the procedure until you've cleaned the entire wound.
- Dry the wound with 4″ × 4″ gauze pads, using the same procedure as for cleaning. Discard the used gauze pads in the plastic trash bag.
- Measure the perimeter of the wound with a disposable wound-measuring device (for example, a square, transparent card with concentric circles arranged in bull's-eye fashion and bordered with a straight-edged ruler). Measure the longest length and the widest width.
- Measure the depth of a full-thickness wound. Insert a sterile cotton-tipped applicator gently into the deepest part of the wound bed and place a mark on the applicator where it meets the skin level. Measure the marked applicator to determine wound depth.

Testing for tunneling
- Gently probe the wound bed and edges with your gloved finger or a sterile cotton-tipped applicator to assess for wound tunneling or undermining. Tunneling usually signals wound extension along fascial planes. Gauge tunnel depth by determining how far you can

insert your gloved finger or the cotton-tipped applicator.

■ Next, reassess the condition of the skin and wound. Note the character of the clean wound bed and the surrounding skin.

■ If you observe adherent necrotic material, notify the primary nurse. A wound care specialist may be consulted to ensure appropriate debridement.

■ Prepare to apply the appropriate topical dressing. Instructions for applying topical moist saline gauze, hydrocolloid, transparent, alginate, foam, and hydrogel dressings are given here. (See *Choosing a wound dressing.*)

For other dressings or topical drugs, follow your facility's protocol or the manufacturer's instructions.

Applying a moist saline gauze dressing

■ Moisten the gauze dressing with normal saline solution. Squeeze out excess fluid.

■ Gently place the dressing into the wound surface. To separate surfaces within the wound, gently guide the gauze between opposing wound surfaces. To avoid damage to tissues, don't pack the gauze tightly.

■ To protect the surrounding skin from moisture, apply a sealant or barrier.

■ Change the dressing often enough to keep the wound moist.

Applying a hydrocolloid dressing

■ Choose a clean, dry, presized dressing, or cut one to overlap the wound by about 1″ (2.5 cm). Remove the dressing from its package, pull the release paper from the adherent side of the dressing, and apply the dressing to the wound. Hold the dressing in place with your hand (the warmth will mold the dressing to the skin).

Choosing a wound dressing

The patient's needs and wound characteristics determine the type of dressing to use on a wound.

GAUZE DRESSINGS

Made of absorptive cotton or synthetic fabric, gauze dressings are permeable to water, water vapor, and oxygen and may be impregnated with hydrogel or another agent. When uncertain about which dressing to use, you may apply a gauze dressing moistened in saline solution until a wound specialist recommends definitive treatment.

HYDROCOLLOID DRESSINGS

Hydrocolloid dressings are adhesive, moldable wafers made of a carbohydrate-based material and usually have waterproof backings. They're impermeable to oxygen, water, and water vapor, and most have some absorptive properties.

TRANSPARENT FILM DRESSINGS

Transparent film dressings are clear, adherent, and nonabsorptive. These polymer-based dressings are permeable to oxygen and water vapor but not to water. Their transparency allows visual inspection. Because they can't absorb drainage, they're used on partial-thickness wounds with minimal exudate.

ALGINATE DRESSINGS

Made from seaweed, alginate dressings are nonwoven, absorptive dressings available as soft white sterile pads or ropes. They absorb excessive exudate and may be used on infected wounds. As these dressings absorb exudate, they turn into a gel that keeps the wound bed moist and promotes healing. When exudate is no longer excessive, switch to another type of dressing.

FOAM DRESSINGS

Foam dressings are spongelike polymer dressings that may be impregnated or coated with other materials. Somewhat absorptive, they may be adherent. These dressings promote moist wound healing and are useful when a nonadherent surface is desired.

(continued)

Choosing a wound dressing (*continued*)

HYDROGEL DRESSINGS
Water-based and nonadherent, hydrogel dressings are polymer-based dressings that have some absorptive properties. They're available as a gel in a tube, as flexible sheets, and as saturated gauze packing strips. They may have a cooling effect, which eases pain, and are used when the wound needs moisture.

▪ As you apply the dressing, carefully smooth out wrinkles and avoid stretching the dressing.
▪ If the dressing's edges need to be secured with tape, apply a skin sealant to the intact skin around the wound. After the area dries, tape the dressing to the skin. The sealant protects the skin from tape burns and skin stripping and promotes tape adherence. Avoid using tension or pressure when applying the tape.
▪ Remove your gloves and discard them in the impervious plastic trash bag. Dispose of refuse according to facility policy, and wash your hands.
▪ Change a hydrocolloid dressing every 2 to 7 days as necessary; change it immediately if the patient complains of pain, the dressing no longer adheres, or leakage occurs.

Applying a transparent dressing
▪ Clean and dry the wound as described previously.
▪ Select a dressing to overlap the wound by 1″ to 2″ (2.5 to 5 cm).
▪ Gently lay the dressing over the wound; avoid wrinkling the dressing. To prevent shearing force, don't stretch the dressing over the wound. Press firmly on the edges of the dressing to promote adherence. Al-

though this type of dressing is self-adhesive, you may have to tape the edges to prevent them from curling.

■ Change the dressing every 3 to 5 days, depending on the amount of drainage. If the seal is no longer secure or if accumulated tissue fluid extends beyond the edges of the wound and onto the surrounding skin, change the dressing.

Applying an alginate dressing

■ Apply the alginate dressing to the wound surface. Cover the area with a secondary dressing (such as gauze pads or transparent film) as ordered. Secure the dressing with tape or elastic netting.

■ If the wound is draining heavily, change the dressing once or twice daily for the first 3 to 5 days. As drainage decreases, change the dressing less frequently—every 2 to 4 days or as ordered. When the drainage stops or the wound bed looks dry, stop using alginate dressing.

Applying a foam dressing

■ Gently lay the foam dressing over the wound.
■ Use tape, elastic netting, or gauze to hold the dressing in place.
■ Change the dressing when the foam no longer absorbs exudate.

Applying a hydrogel dressing

■ Apply a moderate amount of gel to the wound bed.
■ Cover the area with a secondary dressing (gauze, transparent film, or foam).
■ Change the dressing daily or as needed to keep the wound bed moist.
■ If the hydrogel dressing you select comes in sheet form, cut the dressing to overlap the wound by 1″ (2.5 cm); then apply as you would a hydrocolloid dressing.

■ Hydrogel dressings also come in a prepackaged, saturated gauze for wounds with cavities that require "dead space" to be filled. Follow the manufacturer's directions.

COMPLICATIONS
■ Infection may cause foul-smelling drainage, persistent pain, severe erythema, induration, and elevated skin and body temperatures. Some dressing and topical agents, however, may also cause an odor.
■ Advancing infection or cellulitis can lead to septicemia. Severe erythema may signal worsening cellulitis, which means the offending organisms have invaded the tissue and are no longer localized.

Wound irrigation

Irrigation cleans tissues and flushes cell debris and drainage from an open wound. It also helps prevent premature surface healing over an abscess pocket or infected tract.

After irrigation, pack open wounds to absorb additional drainage. Always follow the standard precaution guidelines of the Centers for Disease Control and Prevention (CDC).

EQUIPMENT
■ Waterproof trash bag
■ Linen-saver pad
■ Emesis basin
■ Clean gloves
■ Sterile gloves, if indicated per facility policy
■ Goggles
■ Gown, if indicated

- Prescribed irrigant such as sterile normal saline solution
- Sterile water or normal saline solution
- Soft rubber or plastic catheter
- Sterile container
- Materials needed for wound care
- Sterile irrigation and dressing set
- Commercial wound cleaner
- 35-ml piston syringe with 19G needle or catheter
- Skin protectant wipe (skin sealant) or other protective skin barrier

PREPARATION

Assemble equipment in the patient's room. Check the expiration date on each sterile package and inspect for tears.

Don't use a solution that has been open longer than 24 hours. As needed, dilute the prescribed irrigant to the correct proportions with sterile water or normal saline solution. Allow the solution to reach room temperature, or warm it to 90° to 95° F (32.2° to 35° C).

Open the waterproof trash bag; place it near the patient's bed. Form a cuff by turning down the top of the trash bag.

IMPLEMENTATION

- Try to coordinate wound irrigation with the practitioner's visit so that he can inspect the wound.
- Check the practitioner's order, assess the patient's condition, and identify allergies. Explain the procedure to the patient, provide privacy, and position the patient correctly for the procedure. Place the linen-saver pad under the patient and place the emesis basin below the wound so that the irrigating solution flows from the wound into the basin.
- Wash your hands, and put on a gown and gloves.

■ Remove the soiled dressing; then discard the dressing and gloves in the trash bag.

■ Establish a clean or sterile field with all the equipment and supplies you'll need for wound irrigation and dressing. Pour the prescribed amount of irrigating solution into a clean or sterile container. Put on a new pair of clean gloves and a gown and goggles, if indicated.

■ Fill the syringe with the irrigating solution and connect the catheter to the syringe. Gently instill a slow, steady stream of solution into the wound until the syringe empties. (See *Irrigating a deep wound.*)

  Make sure the solution reaches all areas of the wound and that it flows from the clean to the dirty area of the wound to prevent contamination of clean tissue by exudate.

■ Refill the syringe, reconnect it to the catheter, and repeat the irrigation. Continue to irrigate the wound until you've administered the prescribed amount of solution or until the solution returns clear. Note the amount of solution administered. Then remove and discard the catheter and syringe in the waterproof trash bag. (See *Wound irrigation tips*, page 90.)

■ Keep the patient positioned to allow further wound drainage into the basin.

■ Clean the area around the wound with normal saline solution and pat dry with gauze; wipe intact surrounding skin with a skin protectant wipe and allow it to dry.

■ Pack the wound lightly and loosely if ordered, and apply a dressing.

■ Remove and discard your gloves and gown.

■ Make sure the patient is comfortable.

■ Dispose of drainage, solutions, trash bag, and soiled equipment and supplies according to facility policy and CDC guidelines.

EXPERT TIPS

Irrigating a deep wound

When preparing to irrigate a wound, attach a 19G catheter to a 35-ml piston syringe. This setup delivers an irrigation pressure of 8 psi, which is effective in cleaning the wound and reducing the risk of trauma and wound infection. To prevent tissue damage or, in an abdominal wound, intestinal perforation, avoid forcing the catheter into the wound.

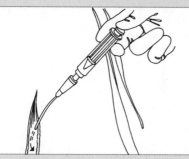

Irrigate the wound with gentle pressure until you've administered the prescribed amount and the solution returns clear. Allow the emesis basin to remain under the wound to collect remaining drainage.

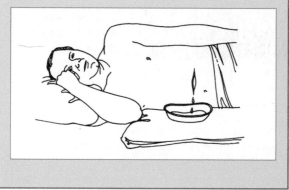

EXPERT TIPS

Wound irrigation tips

How can you avoid mess or spillage when irrigating a wound in a hard-to-reach location? Here are some tips you can follow.

LIMB WOUNDS
An arm or leg wound may be soaked in a large vessel of warm irrigating fluid, such as water, normal saline solution, or an appropriate antiseptic. An agitator can help dislodge bacteria and loosen debris.

If possible, rinse the wound several times and carefully dispose of the contaminated liquid. Reserve the equipment you used for that particular patient. Dry and store it after soaking it in disinfectant. Remember, never soak a limb if the patient has cellulitis, deep vein thrombosis, or other contraindications to soaking in warm water.

TRUNK OR THIGH WOUNDS
Because they're difficult to irrigate, trunk or thigh wounds require some ingenuity. One device uses Stomahesive and a plastic irrigating chamber applied over the wound. (Run warm solution through an infusion set and collect it in a drainage bag.)

A syringe irrigation is another alternative. Where possible, direct the flow at right angles to the wound and allow the fluid to drain by gravity. Doing so requires careful positioning of the patient, either in bed or on a chair. The patient may need analgesia during the treatment.

If irrigation isn't possible, you'll have to swab clean the wound, which is time-consuming. Swab away exudate before using antiseptic or saline solution to clean the wound (taking care not to push loose debris into the wound).

■ If the wound is small or not particularly deep or if a piston syringe is unavailable, irrigate with a bulb syringe. However, use a bulb syringe cautiously because this type of syringe doesn't deliver enough pressure to adequately clean the wound.

Debridement

Debridement of nonviable tissue is the most important factor in wound management. Wound healing can't take place until necrotic tissue is removed. Necrotic tissue may present as moist yellow or gray tissue that's separating from viable tissue. If this moist, necrotic tissue becomes dry, it presents as thick, hard, leathery black eschar. Areas of necrotic tissue may mask underlying fluid collections or abscesses. Although debridement can be painful (especially with burns), it's necessary to prevent infection and promote healing of burns and other wounds.

TYPES OF DEBRIDEMENT

Debridement of necrotic tissue may be accomplished by sharp, autolytic, chemical, or mechanical techniques.

Sharp debridement

Sharp debridement, which is categorized as either conservative or surgical, involves removing necrotic tissue from the wound bed with the use of a cutting tool, such as a scalpel, scissors, or a laser. Conservative sharp debridement involves the removal of necrotic tissue only and is usually done by a practitioner licensed to do so. Surgical sharp debridement involves the removal of both necrotic and healthy tissue, converting a chronic wound to a clean, acute wound. Surgical sharp debridement is typically beyond the practice of nonphysician providers. Caution should be used when providing either conservative or surgical sharp debridement on patients who have low platelet counts or who are taking anticoagulants.

Conservative sharp debridement of a wound involves careful prying and cutting of loosened eschar with forceps and scissors to separate it from viable tissue beneath. One of the most painful types of debridement, it may require either topical or systemic analgesic administration before performing the procedure.

Because you're more likely to be involved in the process of autolytic, chemical, or mechanical debridement, these procedures are covered here in detail.

Autolytic debridement

Autolytic debridement involves the use of moisture-retentive dressings to cover the wound bed. Necrotic tissue is then dissolved through self-digestion of enzymes in the wound fluid. Although autolytic debridement takes longer than other debridement methods, it isn't painful, it's easy to do, and it's appropriate for patients who can't tolerate other methods. If the wound is infected, however, autolytic debridement isn't the treatment of choice.

Chemical debridement

Chemical debridement with enzymatic agents is a selective method of debridement. Enzymes are applied topically to areas of necrotic tissue only, breaking down necrotic tissue elements. These enzymes digest only necrotic tissue—they don't harm healthy tissue. These agents require specific conditions that vary from product to product. Effectiveness is achieved by carefully following each manufacturer's guidelines. Use of the enzymes stops when the wound is clean with red granulation tissue.

Mechanical debridement

Mechanical debridement includes wet-to-dry dressings, irrigation, and hydrotherapy. Wet-to-dry dressings, typically used for wounds with extensive necrotic tissue and minimal drainage, require an appropriate technique and the dressing materials used are critical to the outcome. The nurse or practitioner places a wet dressing in contact with the lesion and covers it with an outer layer of bandaging. As the dressing dries, it sticks to the wound. When the dried dressing is removed, the necrotic tissue comes off with it.

Irrigation of a wound with a pressurized antiseptic solution cleans tissue and removes wound debris and excess drainage.

Hydrotherapy—commonly referred to as *tubbing, tanking,* or *whirlpool*—involves immersing the patient in a tank of warm water, with intermittent agitation of the water. It's usually performed on large wounds with a significant amount of nonviable tissue covering the wound surface, such as with burns.

EQUIPMENT
■ Two pairs of sterile gloves
■ Two gowns or aprons
■ Mask
■ Cap
■ Sterile scissors
■ Sterile forceps
■ Sterile 4″ × 4″ gauze pads
■ Sterile solutions and medications as ordered
■ Hemostatic agent as ordered

Also have the following equipment immediately available to control bleeding.
■ Needle holder
■ Gut suture with needle

IMPLEMENTATION
■ Explain the procedure to the patient to allay his fears and promote cooperation. Teach him distraction and relaxation techniques, if possible, to minimize his discomfort. Acknowledge the patient's discomfort and provide emotional support.

■ Work quickly—with an assistant if possible—to complete this painful procedure as fast as possible. Try to limit procedure time to 20 minutes. Serial debridement may be necessary to rid the wound of necrotic tissue.

■ Provide privacy. Make sure that the patient receives drugs for pain before debridement begins.

Wet-to-dry dressings

■ Put on clean nonsterile gloves.

■ Slowly and gently remove the old dressing, using saline solution to moisten portions of the dressing that don't easily pull away. Discard the old dressing and gloves in a waterproof trash bag.

■ Put on clean gloves.

■ Using sterile technique, moisten an open-weave cotton gauze dressing with saline solution and loosely pack it into the wound. Make sure the entire wound surface is lightly covered with moistened gauze.

■ Apply an outer dressing and secure it with tape or an adhesive bandage.

■ Remove the dressing after it completely dries and becomes adherent to the necrotic tissue (typically in 4 to 6 hours).

Irrigation

■ Use sterile technique to instill a slow, steady stream of solution into the wound with an irrigating syringe or catheter. (For more information, see the irrigation procedure earlier in this chapter.)

Hydrotherapy

■ Prepare the tub, and obtain the patient's vital signs.

■ Put on clean gloves, remove the patient's dressing, and discard all items in a waterproof trash bag.

■ Assist the patient into the tub.
■ After the patient or limb has been immersed in the swirling water for the prescribed amount of time (10 to 20 minutes), spray rinse and pat dry the patient before reapplying sterile dressings.

Sharp debridement
■ Keep the patient warm. Expose only the area to be debrided to prevent chilling and fluid and electrolyte loss.
■ Wash your hands, and put on clean gloves.
■ Remove the wound dressings and clean the wound.
■ Remove your dirty gloves and change into sterile gloves to assist the practitioner.
■ The practitioner will lift loosened edges of eschar with sterile forceps and cut the dead tissue from the wound with the scissors.
■ Irrigate the wound after the procedure, as ordered.
■ Because debridement removes only dead tissue, bleeding should be minimal. If bleeding occurs, apply gentle pressure on the wound with sterile 4″ × 4″ gauze pads. If bleeding persists, notify the practitioner and maintain pressure on the wound. Excessive bleeding or spurting vessels may warrant ligation.
■ Perform additional procedures, such as application of topical medications and dressing replacements, as ordered.

Wound specimen collection

Wound specimen collection involves using a sterile cotton-tipped swab, aspiration with a syringe, or punch tissue biopsy to help identify pathogens.

Because most wounds are colonized with surface bacteria, the swab specimen technique is limited in that it only obtains surface cultures. Needle aspiration of fluid or punch tissue biopsy is recommended for accurate wound culturing. These techniques are performed by practitioners, physician assistants, advanced practice nurses, or certified wound specialists.

EQUIPMENT
- Sterile gloves
- Alcohol pads or povidone-iodine pads
- Sterile swabs
- Sterile 10-ml syringe
- Sterile 21G needle
- Sterile culture tube with transport medium (or commercial collection kit for aerobic culture)
- Labels
- Special anaerobic culture tube containing carbon dioxide or nitrogen
- Fresh dressings for the wound
- Laboratory request form
- Patient labels
- *Optional:* Rubber stopper for needle

IMPLEMENTATION
- Note recent antibiotic therapy on the laboratory request form.
- Although you would normally clean the area around a wound to prevent contamination by normal skin flora, don't clean a perineal wound with alcohol because this could irritate sensitive tissues. Make sure that antiseptic doesn't enter the wound.
- Provide privacy and explain the procedure to the patient.
- Wash your hands, prepare a sterile field, and put on sterile gloves.
- Remove the dressing to expose the wound.
- Dispose of the soiled dressings properly.

- Clean the wound well.
- Inspect the wound, noting the color, amount, and odor of drainage and presence of necrotic debris.
- Clean the area around the wound with an alcohol pad or a povidone-iodine pad to reduce the risk of contaminating the specimen with skin bacteria.
- Allow the area to dry.

Aerobic culture

- Compress the edges of the wound to elicit new drainage.
- Rotate a sterile cotton-tipped swab on the sides and base of the wound bed. If the wound is dry, dip the swab into the transport medium to moisten the tip before swabbing the base of the wound.
- Remove the swab from the wound, and immediately place it in the aerobic culture tube.
- Label the culture tube and send the tube to the laboratory immediately with a completed laboratory request form.
- Never collect exudate from the skin and then insert the same swab into the wound; this could contaminate the wound with skin bacteria.

Anaerobic culture

- Obtain a wound fluid sample as described previously. Immediately place it in the anaerobic culture tube. (See *Anaerobic specimen collector,* page 98.)
- Alternatively, insert a sterile 10-ml syringe, without a needle, into the wound, and aspirate 1 to 5 ml of exudate into the syringe. Then attach the 21G needle to the syringe, and immediately inject the aspirate into the anaerobic culture tube.
- If an anaerobic culture tube is unavailable, obtain a rubber stopper, attach the needle to the syringe, and gently push all the air out of the syringe by pressing on

Anaerobic specimen collector

Because most anaerobes die when exposed to oxygen, they must be transported in tubes filled with carbon dioxide or nitrogen. The anaerobic specimen collector shown here includes a tube filled with carbon dioxide, a small inner tube, and a swab attached to a plastic plunger.

Before specimen collection, the small inner tube containing the swab is held in place with the rubber stopper (shown below left). After collecting the specimen, quickly replace the swab in the inner tube and depress the plunger to separate the inner tube from the stopper (shown below right), forcing it into the larger tube and exposing the specimen to a carbon dioxide–rich environment.

BEFORE   **AFTER**

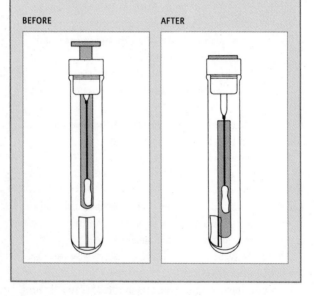

the plunger. Stick the needle tip into the rubber stopper, remove and discard your gloves, and send the syringe of aspirate to the laboratory immediately with a completed laboratory request form.

5

ACUTE WOUNDS

Three factors are used to classify wounds and determine wound severity: age, depth, and color. Wound age is typically described as acute or chronic, which seems simple enough until you ask, "At what point does an acute wound become a chronic wound?" Time alone isn't the distinguishing factor. Progress toward complete healing is also a component. Therefore, an acute wound is better characterized by these criteria:

- It's a new or relatively new wound.
- It occurred suddenly (as opposed to developing over time).
- Healing is progressing in a timely, predictable, and measurable manner.

Acute wounds can occur by intention or trauma. A surgical incision is an example of an acute wound that's caused intentionally. Traumatic wounds can range from simple to severe. Burns are a category of traumatic wound that have a unique set of causes, potential complications, and treatment options, so we'll look at them separately.

Regardless of the cause, caring for a patient with an acute wound focuses on restoring normal anatomic structure, physiologic function, and appearance to the wound area.

Surgical wounds

An acute surgical wound is a healthy and uncomplicated break in the skin's continuity resulting from surgery. In an otherwise healthy individual, this type of wound responds well to postoperative care and heals without incident in a predictable period of time.

FACTORS THAT AFFECT HEALING

Several factors can greatly affect the course of postoperative healing. These include the patient's age, nutritional status, general health before surgery, preexisting illness or infection, and oxygenation status.

Age

Age is an important factor in the healing process, especially for children and older adults. In a premature infant, for example, the immune system and other body systems aren't fully developed; thus, he's at greater risk for infection before, during, and after surgery. Sterile technique is a critical component of care for such patients.

At the other end of the age continuum, older adults commonly have a harder time healing after surgery because of skin changes. As a person ages, skin becomes thinner and less elastic. The cells that repair tissues and fight infection decline in number, and the skin's vascular system is less robust. As a result, surgical wounds in older patients heal more slowly, increasing the risk of infection.

Nutrition

Proper nutrition is crucial for the body to heal itself effectively. During your care of the patient, it's imperative that you identify nutritional problems early and help develop a plan that addresses deficits.

After surgery, the body quickly depletes its stores of nutrients and an otherwise healthy patient can become malnourished if diet is ignored. The patient's diet should include adequate nutrients to maintain homeostasis and create an optimum environment for wound healing.

A patient who's overweight has an additional problem. Adipose tissue lacks the extensive vascular supply present in skin. As the amount of adipose tissue increases, blood flow to the skin decreases, reducing the amount of oxygen and nutrients reaching the area of the wound and impeding healing. An increase in the amount of adipose tissue also places the patient at higher risk for dehiscence.

Illness or infection

In most cases, a preexisting illness or infection delays or complicates healing after surgery. Unfortunately, it isn't always possible to delay surgery until an underlying condition resolves itself. In these cases, care must include measures that minimize the impact of the preexisting condition on the healing process. (See *Minimizing the impact of preexisting conditions on the healing process*, page 102.)

Signs of wound infection include:
■ increased exudate
■ purulent (pus-containing) exudate
■ erythema (reddened tissue) around the wound
■ warmer skin temperature at or around the wound
■ new or increased pain
■ general malaise
■ fever
■ high white blood cell count.

All open wounds are colonized with surface bacteria, but infected wounds are slow to heal and may become dehisced or eviscerated.

Minimizing the impact of preexisting conditions on the healing process

- Disorders that impede blood flow, such as coronary artery disease, peripheral vascular disease, and hypertension, can cause problems by reducing the flow of blood reaching the incision site. A patient with one of these conditions requires patient care that includes interventions to improve circulation.

- Cancer may necessitate more aggressive pain management or patient care that includes management of such symptoms as nausea and vomiting.

- Diabetes mellitus impedes healing in many ways and increases the patient's risk of infection. If present, diabetic neuropathy (inflammation and degeneration of peripheral nerves) may interfere with vasodilation and, consequently, circulation in the area of the incision. Hyperglycemia generally lengthens the healing time.

- Immunosuppression resulting from either a disease or drug therapy (corticosteroids, chemotherapy) may impair the inflammatory response, delaying wound healing and increasing the patient's risk of infection.

- Care should focus on keeping the wound clean and protecting it from trauma.

Oxygenation status

During healing, neutrophils require oxygen to produce the hydrogen peroxide they use to kill pathogens, and fibroblasts require oxygen for collagen proliferation; therefore, adequate oxygenation is critical to the healing process. A condition that impedes overall oxygenation or the amount of oxygen reaching the wound—atherosclerosis, for example—slows the healing process.

PATIENT CARE

Proper care during healing varies depending on the method of wound closure used, the development of the healing ridge, and the type of dressing indicated. The patient's ability to properly perform wound care after discharge also affects healing.

Wound closure

The surgeon determines the appropriate method of wound closure based on the wound's severity; in many cases, sutures are used.

In suturing, a natural or synthetic thread is used to stitch the wound closed. (See *Types of suture materials and methods,* pages 104 and 105.)

Sutures typically remain in place for 7 to 10 days, depending on the severity of the wound and the type of tissue involved, provided that healing is progressing as expected. Factors that affect the timing of suture removal include the patient's overall condition; the shape, size, and location of the incision; and whether inflammation, drainage, dehiscence, or infection develops.

The surgeon may choose to use skin staples or clips as an alternative to sutures if cosmetic results aren't an issue. These closures secure a wound faster than sutures and, because they're made of surgical stainless steel, tissue reaction is reduced. Properly placed staples and clips distribute tension evenly along the suture line, reducing tissue trauma and compression. This promotes healing and minimizes scarring. The surgeon won't use staples or clips if less than 5 mm of tissue exists between the staple and underlying bone, vessel, or organ.

Smaller wounds with little drainage can be closed with adhesive skin closures, such as Steri-Strips or butterfly closures. As with staples and clips, these closures cause

Types of suture materials and methods

When closing a surgical wound, the choice of suture material varies according to the suturing method, location, and tissue type.

MATERIALS

Nonabsorbable sutures are used to close the skin surface. They provide strength and immobility and minimize tissue irritation. Nonabsorbable suture materials include silk, cotton, stainless steel, and Dacron.

When suture removal is undesirable—for example, sutures in an underlying tissue layer—the surgeon may choose an *absorbable suture.* Absorbable suture materials include:

● chromic catgut—a natural catgut treated with chromium trioxide to improve strength and prolong absorption time

● plain catgut—a material that's absorbed faster and is more likely to cause irritation than chromic catgut

● synthetic materials—materials such as polyglycolic acid that are replacing catgut because they're stronger, more durable, and less irritating.

METHODS

The most common suture methods include mattress continuous suture, plain continu-ous suture, mattress interrupted suture, plain interrupted suture, and blanket continuous suture. These methods are described here.

MATTRESS CONTINUOUS SUTURE

Mattress continuous suture is a series of connected mattress stitches with a knot at the beginning and end.

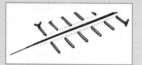

PLAIN CONTINUOUS SUTURE

Also called a *continuous running suture,* a plain continuous suture is a series of connected stitches. The thread is knotted at the beginning and at the end of the suture.

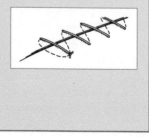

Types of suture materials and methods
(continued)

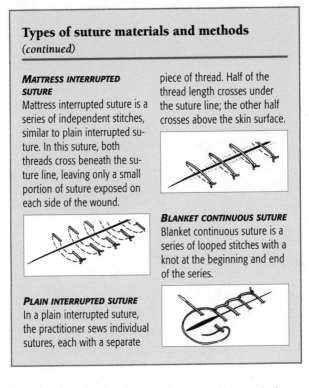

MATTRESS INTERRUPTED SUTURE
Mattress interrupted suture is a series of independent stitches, similar to plain interrupted suture. In this suture, both threads cross beneath the suture line, leaving only a small portion of suture exposed on each side of the wound.

piece of thread. Half of the thread length crosses under the suture line; the other half crosses above the skin surface.

BLANKET CONTINUOUS SUTURE
Blanket continuous suture is a series of looped stitches with a knot at the beginning and end of the series.

PLAIN INTERRUPTED SUTURE
In a plain interrupted suture, the practitioner sews individual sutures, each with a separate

little tissue reaction. Adhesive closures can be used after suture or staple removal to provide ongoing support for a healing incision. (See *Types of adhesive skin closures,* page 106.)

The healing ridge
To properly assess healing, it's important to understand how the healing ridge develops in an incision after surgery. The healing ridge is a buildup of collagen fibers that begins to form during the inflammatory phase of wound healing (usually the first 24 to 72 hours) and peaks during the proliferation phase (about days 5 to 9). You

Types of adhesive skin closures

The two most common types of adhesive skin closures are Steri-Strips and butterfly closures.

STERI-STRIPS
Steri-Strips, thin strips of sterile, nonwoven tape, are a primary means of holding a wound closed after suture removal.

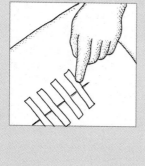

BUTTERFLY CLOSURES
Butterfly closures have two sterile, waterproof adhesive strips connected by a narrow, nonadhesive "bridge." These strips are used to hold small wounds closed to promote healing after suture removal.

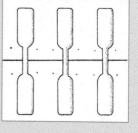

should feel this ridge as you gently palpate the skin on each side of the wound. The healing ridge is a sign that healing is progressing. If you can't feel this ridge, healing isn't progressing as expected, further assessment is required, and the primary nurse and surgeon should be notified. When the ridge fails to develop, mechanical strain on the wound is most likely at fault, and the wound is at a higher risk of dehiscence.

Dressings
The incision dressing shields the wound against pathogens and should protect the skin surface from irritating drainage. The dressing is the primary aspect of wound

management for surgical wounds, so choosing the correct type is important.

Typically, lightly exuding wounds with drains and wounds with minimal purulent drainage require only loose packing and a gauze dressing. A wound with copious, excoriating drainage requires an absorbent dressing such as an alginate or pouching to contain the drainage and protect the surrounding skin. (See *Pouching a wound,* pages 108 and 109.) When dressing a surgical wound, use sterile technique and sterile supplies to prevent contamination. Change the dressing as often as needed to absorb drainage and keep the surrounding skin dry. Remember, however, that a wound heals best at body temperature; changing the dressing lowers the temperature at the wound site and healing slows until the site returns to normal body temperature.

PATIENT EDUCATION

Patient education is an important care plan component for patients with surgical wounds. By the time he's discharged, the patient needs to understand—and demonstrate—the ability to perform proper wound care. Start with a determination of the patient's knowledge. Then begin teaching with a discussion of basic asepsis and handwashing techniques. The balance of your teaching depends on the type of surgery, the type of dressing, the frequency of dressing changes or care, and the location of the wound. (See *Teaching about surgical wound care,* page 110.)

POTENTIAL COMPLICATIONS

Surgery results in a controlled form of acute wound. The patient's environment, the type and severity of the wound, and preoperative and postoperative care are all under the control of members of the health care team. Consequently,

EXPERT TIPS

Pouching a wound

If your patient's wound is draining heavily or if drainage may damage surrounding skin, you need to apply a pouch. Here's how:

● Measure the wound. Cut an opening ⅜" larger than the wound in the facing of the collection pouch (see photo below).

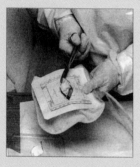

● Apply a skin protectant as needed. (Some protectants are incorporated into the collection pouch system and also provide adhesion.)
● Be sure to close the drainage port at the bottom of the pouch to prevent leaks. Then gently press the contoured pouch opening around the wound, starting at the lower edge, to catch any drainage (see photo top of next column).

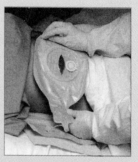

● To empty the pouch, put on gloves, a face shield or mask, and eye protection. Insert the lower portion of the pouch into a graduated biohazard container and open the drainage port (see photo top of next page).
● Note the color, consistency, odor, and amount of fluid. If ordered, obtain a culture specimen and send it to the laboratory immediately. Always follow Centers for Disease Control and Prevention standard precautions when handling infectious drainage.

Pouching a wound *(continued)*

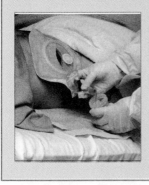

● Use a gauze pad to wipe the bottom of the pouch and the drainage port. This prevents skin irritation or possible odor from any residual drainage. Reseal the port.
● Change the pouch only if it leaks or fails to adhere. More frequent changes are unnecessary and can irritate the patient's skin.

most surgical wounds heal without incident. Some complications that might arise, however, include wound infection, hemorrhage, and wound dehiscence or evisceration.

Wound infection

Wound infection is the most common wound complication and the second most common hospital-acquired infection. Preventing wound infection requires meticulous attention to sterile technique when caring for an acute wound.

For a surgical patient, wound infection is a significant and serious event requiring prompt intervention. Interventions typically indicated in cases of postoperative infection include:

■ obtaining a wound culture and sensitivity test
■ giving antibiotics
■ irrigating the wound
■ dressing the wound and packing it, if necessary
■ monitoring wound drainage.

Teaching about surgical wound care

Surgical patients need to know the ways they can promote healing and prevent infection. Be sure to discuss:

● signs and symptoms of wound infection that should be reported to the practitioner immediately, such as increased tenderness, deep or increased pain at the wound site, fever, or edema (especially if it occurs between postoperative days 3 and 5)
● the way to obtain an accurate temperature reading
● proper wound care, such as the importance of keeping the incision clean and dry; proper hand-washing technique; and the supplies and methods used to clean the wound
● wound dressings, including the type, proper application methods, and places to obtain them
● types and levels of permissible activity, such as when the patient may shower or bathe, restrictions on lifting (if applicable), when the patient may resume driving, and when the patient can expect to return to work
● follow-up appointments.

Hemorrhage

Hemorrhage may occur from damage to blood vessels. In the postoperative patient, it may happen in either internal or external sites.

The most common locations of significant internal hemorrhages are the posterior nasal passages, pulmonary vessels, spleen, liver, stomach, and uterus. Hemorrhage may also occur at the site of a large artery injury or aneurysm. Hemorrhage in one of these areas significantly reduces the volume of circulating blood and precipitates hypovolemia. Nursing interventions include giving I.V. fluids to increase blood pressure and urine output and helping determine the source of bleeding.

If the hemorrhage originates externally—for example, from the wound itself or from damage to the fragile, newly developed blood vessels—place pressure or a pressure dressing on the site of the bleeding and notify the primary nurse and surgeon for specific treatments.

Wound dehiscence and evisceration

Dehiscence is most likely to occur when collagen fibers aren't mature enough to hold the incision closed without sutures. The first sign of dehiscence may be a gush of serosanguineous fluid from the wound or a report from the patient of a popping sensation after sneezing, coughing, or retching. Complete dehiscence leads to evisceration, in which underlying tissues protrude through the wound opening. Abdominal wounds are more likely to dehisce and eviscerate than thoracic wounds.

To prevent wound dehiscence and evisceration, teach the patient to support the incision with a pillow or cushion before he changes position, coughs, or sneezes.

If dehiscence occurs, take these steps:

- Stay with the patient; keep him still and have a colleague notify the primary nurse and surgeon.
- If the patient has an abdominal wound, help him into low Fowler's position, with knees bent to reduce abdominal tension.
- If evisceration is evident, cover the extruding tissues with sterile abdominal dressings soaked with sterile normal saline solution.

Traumatic wounds

A traumatic wound is a sudden, unplanned injury to the skin that can range from minor (such as a skinned knee) to severe (such as a gunshot wound). This category of wounds includes abrasions, lacerations, skin tears, bites, and penetrating wounds.

Classifying skin tears

The Payne-Martin classification system is a common system used to grade the severity of a skin tear.

CATEGORY I
Skin tears without tissue loss
A. Linear type—epidermis and dermis pulled apart as if an incision has been made
B. Flat type—epidermal flap completely covers the dermis to within 1 mm of the wound margin

CATEGORY II
Skin tears with partial tissue loss
A. Scant tissue-loss type—25% or less of the epidermal flap lost
B. Moderate to large tissue type—more than 25% of the epidermal flap lost

CATEGORY III
Skin tears with complete tissue loss

Adapted with permission from Payne, R.L., and Martin, M.L. "Defining and Classifying Skin Tears: Need for a Common Language," *Ostomy/Wound Management* 39(5):16, June 1993.

ABRASIONS

An abrasion occurs when a mechanical force, such as friction or shearing, scrapes away a partial thickness of the skin. Unless an unusually large amount of skin is involved or an infection develops, an abrasion is one of the least complicated traumatic wounds.

LACERATIONS

A laceration is a tear in the skin that's caused by a sharp object, such as metal, glass, or wood. It can also be caused by trauma that produces high shearing force. A laceration has jagged, irregular edges and its severity depends on its cause, size, depth, and location.

Preventing skin tears

As aging occurs, the skin becomes more susceptible to skin tear injuries. With a little effort and education, you can substantially reduce a patient's risk. Prevent skin tears by:

● using proper lifting, positioning, transferring, and turning techniques to reduce or eliminate friction or shear

● padding support surfaces where risk is greatest, such as bed rails and limb supports on a wheelchair

● using pillows or cushions to support the patient's arms and legs

● telling the patient to add protection by wearing long-sleeved shirts and long pants, as weather permits

● using nonadhering dressings or those with minimal adherent, such as paper tape, and using a skin barrier wipe before applying dressings

● removing tape or other adhesives cautiously, using the push-pull technique

● using wraps, such as a stockinette or soft gauze, to protect areas of skin where the risk of tearing is high

● telling the patient to avoid sudden movements that can pull the skin and possibly cause a skin tear

● applying skin lotion twice per day to areas at risk

● using a significant amount of padding between the skin and a limb restraint, if one is being used.

Skin tears

A skin tear is a specific type of laceration that most often affects older adults. In a skin tear, friction alone—or shearing force plus friction—separates layers of skin. Skin tears are categorized based on the amount of tissue loss. (See *Classifying skin tears*.)

This type of injury may be preventable through careful handling by members of the health care team. (See *Preventing skin tears*.)

BITES

When assessing a bite wound, it's important to quickly discover the bite's source—cat, dog, bat, snake, spider, human, or another animal or insect. This helps the health care team determine which bacteria or toxins may be present and the likely type of tissue trauma.

For example, a human bite can cause a puncture wound and introduce any one of the innumerable organisms present in the human mouth into the wound. *Staphylococcus aureus* and streptococci are two such organisms that can be transmitted to the wound or into the victim's bloodstream. Other serious diseases that can be transmitted in this way include human immunodeficiency virus infection, hepatitis B, hepatitis C, syphilis, and tuberculosis. Some evidence suggests that a human bite can also cause necrotizing fasciitis.

A bite from a dog, cat, or rodent can introduce deadly infectious diseases, such as rabies, into the wound. In terms of tissue damage, cats and other smaller mammals do relatively little damage. However, a dog can generate up to 200 psi of pressure when biting and if he shakes his head at the same time, which is usually the case, strong torsional force can cause a massive amount of tissue damage.

PENETRATING WOUNDS

A penetrating wound is a puncture wound. This type of wound may be the result of an accident or a personal attack, as in the case of a stabbing or gunshot wound.

Stab wounds are low-velocity, penetrating wounds that generally present as classic puncture wounds or lacerations. In some cases, however, they may involve organ damage beneath the site of the wound. X-rays, computed tomography scanning, and magnetic resonance imaging are used to evaluate possible organ damage. If the weapon used is contaminated, the patient should be treated for local infection, sepsis, and tetanus.

A gunshot wound is a high-velocity, penetrating wound. Factors that affect the severity of tissue damage include the caliber of the weapon, the velocity of the projectile, and the patient's position at the time of injury.

In most cases, a small-caliber weapon firing a relatively low-velocity projectile creates a small, clean punctuate lesion with little or no bleeding. If the projectile is no longer in the patient's body, treat this lesion as you would any other open wound.

A large-caliber, relatively high-velocity projectile typically causes massive tissue destruction, a large gaping wound, profuse bleeding, and wound contamination. In this case, the patient usually requires immediate surgical intervention. After surgery, treat the wound as a surgical wound.

PATIENT CARE

Time is critical when caring for a patient with a traumatic wound. First, assess airway, breathing, and circulation (ABCs). Although focusing first on the injury itself may seem natural, a patent airway and pumping heart take priority.

Next, turn your attention to the wound. Control bleeding by applying firm, direct pressure and elevate the patient's extremities. If bleeding continues, you may need to compress a pressure point above the wound. Then assess the wound's condition. Specific wound management and cleaning depend on the type of wound and degree of contamination. (See *Caring for a traumatic wound,* pages 116 and 117.)

Caring for a traumatic wound

When caring for a patient with a traumatic wound, always begin by assessing the ABCs: airway, breathing, and circulation. Move on to the wound itself only after ABCs are stable. Here are the basic steps to follow in caring for each type of traumatic wound.

ABRASION
- Flush the area of the abrasion with normal saline solution or wound cleaning solution.
- Use a sterile 4″ × 4″ gauze pad moistened with normal saline solution to remove dirt or gravel, and gently rub toward the entry point to work contaminants back out the way they entered.
- If the wound is extremely dirty, you may need to scrub it with a surgical brush. Be as gentle as possible and keep in mind that this is a painful process for your patient.
- Allow a small wound to dry and form a scab. Cover larger wounds with a nonadherent pad or petroleum gauze and a light dressing. Apply antibacterial ointment if ordered.

LACERATION
- Moisten a sterile 4″ × 4″ gauze pad with normal saline solution or wound cleaning solution. Gently clean the wound, beginning at the center and working out to approximately 2″ (5 cm) beyond the edge of the wound. Whenever the pad becomes soiled, discard it and use a new one. Continue until the wound appears clean.
- If necessary, irrigate the wound using a 50-ml catheter-tip syringe and normal saline solution.
- Assist the practitioner in suturing the wound if necessary; apply sterile strips of porous tape if suturing isn't needed.
- Apply antibacterial ointment as ordered to prevent infection.
- Apply a dry sterile dressing over the wound to absorb drainage and help prevent bacterial contamination.

BITE
- Immediately irrigate the wound with copious amounts of normal saline solution. Don't immerse and soak the wound; this may allow bacteria to float back into the tissue.

Caring for a traumatic wound (*continued*)

• Clean the wound with sterile 4″ × 4″ gauze pads and an antiseptic such as povidone-iodine.
• Assist with debridement if indicated.
• Apply a loose dressing. If the bite is on an extremity, elevate it to reduce swelling.
• Ask the patient about the animal that bit him to determine whether there's a risk of rabies. Administer rabies and tetanus shots as needed.

PENETRATING WOUND
• If the wound is minor, allow it to bleed for a few minutes before cleaning it. A larger puncture wound may require irrigation.
• Cover the wound with a dry dressing.
• If the wound contains an embedded foreign object, such as a shard of glass or metal, stabilize the object until the practitioner can remove it. When the object is removed and bleeding is under control, clean the wound as you would a laceration.
• Administer tetanus, as needed.

SPECIAL CONSIDERATIONS

In caring for a patient with a traumatic wound, pay particular attention to these aspects of care:

■ When irrigating the wound, avoid using more than 8 psi of pressure. High-pressure irrigation can seriously interfere with healing by destroying cells and forcing bacteria into the tissue.

■ When cleaning the wound, use sterile normal saline solution to remove debris. Never instill hydrogen peroxide into a deep wound—the evolving gases can cause an embolism.

■ Avoid using alcohol to clean a traumatic wound. It's painful for the patient and it dehydrates tissue. Avoid cleaning with antiseptics because they can impede healing.

■ Never use a cotton ball or a cotton-filled gauze pad to clean a wound because cotton fibers left in the wound may cause contamination or a foreign body reaction.

■ If the practitioner plans to debride the wound to remove dead tissue and reduce the risk of infection and scarring, loosely pack the wound with gauze pads soaked in normal saline solution until it's time for the procedure.

■ Monitor closely for signs of developing infection, such as warm, red skin or purulent discharge from the wound. Infection in a traumatic wound can delay healing, increase scarring, and trigger systemic infections such as septicemia.

■ Inspect the dressings regularly. If edema develops, adjust the dressing to ensure adequate circulation to the area of the wound.

Burns

A burn is an acute wound caused by exposure to thermal extremes, caustic chemicals, electricity, or radiation. The degree of tissue damage depends on the strength of the source and the duration of contact or exposure.

Thermal burns

Thermal burns, the most common type of burn, can result from virtually any misuse or mishandling of fire or a combustible product. Playing with matches, pouring gasoline into a hot lawnmower, and setting off fireworks are some common examples of ways in which thermal burns occur. Thermal burns can also result from kitchen accidents, house or office fires, automobile accidents, or physical abuse. Although less common, exposure to extreme cold can also cause thermal burns.

Chemical burns
Chemical burns most commonly result from contact (skin contact or inhalation) with a caustic agent, such as an acid, an alkali, or a vesicant.

Electrical burns
Electrical burns result from contact with flowing electrical current. Household current, high-voltage transmission lines, and lightning are sources of electrical burns.

Radiation burns
The most common radiation burn is sunburn, which follows excessive exposure to the sun. Almost all other burns due to radiation exposure occur as a result of radiation treatment or in specific industries that use or process radioactive materials.

ASSESSMENT
Initial assessment should be conducted as soon as possible after the burn occurs. First, assess ABCs. Then determine the patient's level of consciousness and mobility. After this, the burn is assessed for size, depth, and severity.

Determining size
Burn size is expressed as a percentage of total body surface area (BSA). The Rule of Nines and the Lund-Browder Classification are two useful tools for providing reasonably standardized and quick estimates of the percentage of BSA affected. (See *Estimating burn size,* pages 120 and 121.)

Assessment provides a general idea of burn severity. A partial-thickness burn damages the epidermis and part of

Estimating burn size

Because body surface area (BSA) varies with age, different methods are used to estimate burn size in adult and children.

RULE OF NINES
You can quickly estimate the extent of an adult's burn by using the Rule of Nines. This method quantifies BSA in multiples of 9, hence the name. To use this method, mentally transfer the burns on your patient to the body charts. Add the corresponding percentages for each body section burned. Use the total—a rough estimate of burn extent—to calculate initial fluid replacement needs.

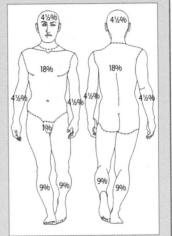

LUND-BROWDER CLASSIFICATION
The Rule of Nines isn't accurate for infants or children because their body shapes, and therefore BSA, differ from those of adults. For example, an infant's head accounts for about 17% of his total BSA, compared with 9% for an adult. Instead, use the Lund- Browder Classification to determine burn size for infants and children.

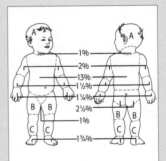

Estimating burn size *(continued)*

PERCENTAGE OF BURNED BODY SURFACE BY AGE

AT BIRTH	0 TO 1 YEAR	1 TO 4 YEARS	5 TO 9 YEARS	10 TO 15 YEARS	ADULT
A: HALF OF HEAD					
9½%	8½%	6½%	5½%	4½%	3½%
B: HALF OF ONE THIGH					
2¾%	3¼%	4%	4¼%	4½%	4¾%
C: HALF OF ONE LEG					
2½%	2½%	2¾%	3%	3¼%	3½%

the dermis; a full-thickness burn also affects subcutaneous tissue. Traditionally, burns were gauged by degree. Today, however, most assessment findings use degree and depth of tissue damage to describe a burn.

- First-degree: localized injury or destruction to the skin's epidermis by direct contact (chemical spill) or indirect contact (sunlight). The barrier function of the skin remains intact.
- Second-degree superficial partial-thickness: involves destruction to the epidermis and some dermis. Thin-walled, fluid-filled blisters develop within a few minutes of the injury. As the blisters break, the nerve endings become exposed to the air. Because pain and tactile responses remain intact, subsequent treatments are painful. The barrier function of the skin is lost.
- Second-degree deep partial-thickness burn: involves the epidermis and dermis. Blisters develop along with mild to moderate edema and pain. There's less pain than with the second-degree superficial partial-thickness burn because of extensive destruction to the

Visualizing burn depth

The most widely used system of classifying burn depth and severity categorizes them by degree. It's important to remember, however, that most burns involve tissue damage of multiple degrees and thicknesses. This illustration may help you visualize burn damage at the various degrees.

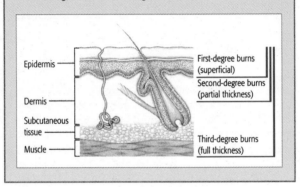

sensory neurons. The barrier function of the skin is lost.

■ Third-degree burn: extends through the epidermis and dermis and into the subcutaneous tissue layer. It may also involve muscle, bone, and interstitial tissue. Fluids and proteins shift from the capillary to the interstitial spaces, causing edema. The body has an immediate immunologic response to a third-degree burn, making burn wound sepsis a potential threat. In most instances, damage involves several depths and degrees. (See *Visualizing burn depth*.)

Determining severity

The severity of a burn is associated with both its size and depth. The three categories of burn severity are major, moderate, and minor.

MAJOR

Major burns meet one or more of these criteria:

- third-degree burns on more than 10% of BSA
- second-degree burns on more than 25% of BSA in adults
- burns on the hands, face, feet, or genitalia
- burns complicated by fractures or respiratory damage
- electrical burns
- any burn in a high-risk patient.

MODERATE

Moderate burns meet one or more of these criteria:

- third-degree burns on 2% to 10% of BSA
- second-degree burns on 15% to 25% of BSA in adults.

MINOR

Minor burns meet one or more of these criteria:

- third-degree burns on less than 2% of BSA
- second-degree burns on less than 15% of BSA in adults.

Special considerations

When caring for a burn victim, pay particular attention to factors that affect treatment and healing, including:

- burn location—burns on the face, hands, feet, and genitalia are most serious due to the possible loss of function
- burn configuration—edema due to a circumferential burn (one that goes completely around an extremity) can slow or stop circulation to the extremity; burns on the neck can obstruct the airway; burns on the chest can interfere with normal respiration by inhibiting expansion

- preexisting medical conditions—note disorders that impair peripheral circulation, especially diabetes, peripheral vascular disease, and chronic alcohol abuse
- other injuries sustained at the time of the burn
- patient age—victims younger than age 4 or older than age 60 are at higher risk for complications and, consequently, for death
- pulmonary injury—inhaling smoke or super-heated air damages lung tissue.

BURN CARE

Care for a burn patient depends on the type and severity of the burn, the patient's general health before the injury, and whether another injury was sustained concurrent with the burn. Treatment seeks to reduce pain; remove dirt, debris, and dead tissue; and provide a dressing that promotes healing. In some cases, treatment includes skin grafting.

If the patient is to be transferred to a burn care unit soon after the accident, wrap him first in a sterile sheet and then a blanket for warmth; elevate the burned extremity to minimize edema.

Minor to moderate burns

In minor to moderate burns, the first step is to stop the burning process and relieve pain. Remove smoldering clothing and give drugs for pain, as indicated. When cleaning a burn, never use hydrogen peroxide or povidone-iodine (or products containing these agents) because they can cause further tissue damage. Cover the burn with dry, sterile towels.

As soon as the patient's condition stabilizes and other injuries are ruled out, the practitioner may order a narcotic analgesic, such as morphine. Be sure to talk to the patient as you work. Emotional support and reassurance are important aspects of care and may reduce the patient's need for analgesia.

After the practitioner debrides devitalized tissue, cover the wound with an antimicrobial and a nonadhesive bulky dressing if needed. Tetanus prophylaxis may be indicated.

Moderate to major burns

In moderate to major burns, immediately assess the patient's ABCs. Be especially alert for signs of smoke inhalation and pulmonary damage—singed nasal hairs, mucosal burns, changes in the patient's voice, coughing, wheezing, soot in the mouth or nose, or darkened sputum. The patient may need endotracheal intubation and 100% oxygen. When the patient's ABCs are stable, a brief history of the burn and blood samples, as ordered, may be obtained.

Next, residual burning must be stopped and bleeding controlled. Remove smoldering clothing. If material is stuck to the patient's skin, soak it with saline solution before attempting to remove it. Remove all jewelry and other constricting items of apparel, then cover the burns with a clean, dry, sterile bed sheet. (Never cover large burns with saline-soaked dressings because this can drastically lower body temperature.)

Monitor I.V. therapy, as indicated per facility policy, to prevent hypovolemic shock and help maintain cardiac output. A patient with serious burns needs massive fluid replacement—especially during the first 24 hours after the injury. At this juncture, the practitioner may order a combination of crystalloids such as lactated Ringer's solution.

Closely monitor the patient's intake and output, and check vital signs often. If the patient's limbs are badly burned, measuring blood pressure can be painful. In order to check blood pressure as required, apply a sterile

Assessing electric shock

When electric current passes through the body, the damage it does depends on the:
- intensity of the current (measured in amperes)
- resistance of the tissues it passes through
- kind of current (alternating current, direct current, or a combination of both)
- frequency and duration of the flow of current.
    Electric current can cause injury in three ways:
- true electrical injury caused by current that passes through the body
- arc or flash burns caused by current that doesn't pass through the body
- thermal surface burns caused by associated heat and flames.
    Prognosis depends on:
- site of the injury
- extent of damage
- patient's general health before the injury
- speed and adequacy of treatment.

nonstick pad to the area first. In addition, be prepared to assist in emergency escharotomy if the patient's burns threaten circulation.

Electrical burns

Tissue damage from electrical burns is difficult to assess because internal damage along the conduction pathway is commonly greater than the surface burn indicates. Knowing the voltage helps the health care team assess possible internal damage more accurately.

Keep in mind that current passing through the body can induce ventricular fibrillation, cardiac arrest, or respiratory arrest—all life-threatening conditions requiring immediate intervention. (See *Assessing electric shock*.)

Chemical burns

When caring for a patient with a chemical burn, irrigate the wound with plenty of sterile water or normal saline solution. Using a weak base, such as sodium bicarbonate, to neutralize an acid spilled on the skin or mucous membranes is controversial, particularly during the emergency phase, because the neutralizing agent can generate more heat, causing additional tissue damage.

If the patient's eyes are involved, flush them with plenty of water or saline solution for at least 30 minutes. If it's an alkaline burn, irrigate until the pH of the conjunctival cul-de-sacs return to 7.0. Then have the patient close his eyes and cover them with dry, sterile dressings. Arrange for an ophthalmologic examination. Lastly, note the type of chemical involved and the presence of noxious fumes.

Skin grafting

Skin grafting may be necessary to repair defects caused by burns, trauma, or surgery. Depending on the graft's complexity, the procedure may be performed under local or general anesthesia and, in some cases, may be performed as an outpatient procedure. (For information on temporary skin grafts, see *Learning about biological dressings,* page 128.)

The surgeon may choose skin grafting as the preferred treatment option if:

■ primary closure isn't possible or cosmetically acceptable
■ primary closure would interfere with function
■ the wound is on a weight-bearing surface of the body
■ a skin tumor is excised and the site needs to be monitored for recurrence.

Learning about biological dressings

Biological dressings function much like skin grafts, preventing infection and fluid loss and easing patient discomfort. Biological dressings are only temporary measures because the body eventually rejects them. If the underlying wound hasn't healed, the dressing must be replaced with a graft of the patient's own skin.

Here's a comparison of the four types of biological dressings and their uses.

TYPE AND SOURCE	USE AND DURATION	SPECIAL CONSIDERATIONS
AMNION Made from amnion and chorionic membranes	Used to protect burns and to temporarily cover granulation tissue awaiting a graft. Must be changed every 48 hours.	● Apply only to clean wounds. ● Leave open to the air or cover with a dressing.
BIOSYNTHETIC Woven from man-made fibers	Used to cover donor sites; to protect clean, superficial burns and excised wounds awaiting grafts; and to cover meshed grafts. Must be reapplied every 3 to 4 days.	● Don't remove to treat the wound (biosynthetic dressings are permeable to antimicrobials).
HETEROGRAFT (XENOGRAFT) Harvested from animals (usually pigs)	Used to protect granulation tissue after escharotomy, to protect excisions, to serve as a test graft before skin grafting, and to temporarily cover burns when the patient doesn't have sufficient skin for immediate grafting. Also used to cover meshed grafts, to protect exposed tendons, and to cover burns that are eschar-free and only slightly contaminated. Usually rejected in 7 to 10 days.	● Dress or leave open. ● Watch for signs of rejection.
HOMOGRAFT (ALLOGRAFT) Harvested from cadavers	Used for same purposes as a heterograft. Usually rejected in 7 to 10 days.	● Observe wound for exudate. ● Watch for local and systemic signs of rejection.

The three types of skin grafts are:

- split-thickness grafts, which consist of the epidermis and a small portion of the dermis
- full-thickness grafts, which include the epidermis and all of the dermis
- composite grafts, which include the epidermis, dermis, and underlying tissues, such as muscle, cartilage, and bone.

The success or failure of a skin graft hinges on revascularization. Initially, a skin graft survives by direct contact with the underlying tissue, receiving oxygen and nutrients through existing blood vessels. The graft dies, however, unless new blood vessels develop. For split-thickness grafts, revascularization usually takes 3 to 5 days; for full-thickness grafts, up to 2 weeks.

PATIENT PREPARATION

A skin graft is taken, or harvested, from an area of healthy tissue on the patient's body. Therefore, it's important to provide meticulous skin care to preserve potential donor sites. Also, because graft survival depends on close contact with underlying tissue, the recipient site—the wound—should be healthy granulation tissue that's free from eschar, debris, and infection.

AFTERCARE

After a skin graft, care focuses on promoting graft survival. Help the patient find comfortable positions for relaxing and sleeping that prevent him from lying on the area of the graft. If feasible, keep the graft elevated and immobilized. When needed, modify your care routine to accommodate healing. For example, never use a blood pressure cuff over a graft site. In the case of a burn patient, omit hydrotherapy until the graft heals. Make sure that the patient receives analgesics as needed, but also teach the patient other techniques, such as breathing and relaxation exercises, to reduce pain without drugs.

Always use sterile technique when changing dressings, and work gently to avoid dislodging the graft. Clean the graft site with a warm saline solution and cotton-tipped applicators, leaving the fine-mesh gauze over the graft intact. Aspirate serous pockets. Change the gauze, apply the prescribed topical agent as indicated, and then cover the area with a gauze bandage.

As the patient prepares to go home, discuss proper wound care with him. Explain that the dressings on the graft and donor sites shouldn't be disturbed for any reason. If he feels the dressing needs to be changed, he should call the practitioner and never attempt it himself. Emphasize that immobilizing the area of the graft is essential for speedy and complete healing. Later, as healing progresses, he can apply cream to the graft site several times per day to keep the skin pliable and help the scar mature.

Sun exposure can affect graft pigmentation. Explain this to your patient and suggest that he limit the amount of time he spends in the sun. Also suggest that he use sunblock anytime he plans to be outdoors.

Lastly, almost all patients express concern about scarring and appearance. If your patient is worried, explain that if scarring continues to be a problem when the graft completely heals, he can discuss plastic surgery options with his practitioner.

6

VASCULAR ULCERS

The vascular system is composed of arteries, veins, capillaries, and lymphatics. Pressure from the beating heart carries blood away from the heart through the arteries into progressively smaller vessels until they connect with the capillaries. On the other side of the capillaries, small veins receive blood and pass it into progressively larger veins on its return trip to the heart. The lymphatic system is a separate system of vessels that collect waste products and deliver them to the venous system.

A group of disorders that affect the blood vessels outside the heart, or the lymphatic vessels, are known collectively as peripheral vascular disease (PVD). Vascular ulcers are acute or chronic wounds that stem from PVD in the venous, arterial, and lymphatic systems. Venous and arterial ulcers are most common in the lower legs and feet, whereas lymphatic ulcers occur in the arms or the legs.

Venous ulcers

Venous ulcers, which result from venous hypertension, occur in the lower leg. They affect about 1% of the population as a whole but are most common in older adults, affecting 3.5% of those older than age 65. Venous ulcers account for 70% to 90% of all leg ulcers.

VENOUS ANATOMY AND FUNCTION

In the circulatory system, arteries carry blood away from the heart, and veins carry blood back to the heart. Capillaries connect these two systems. On the venous side, venules are the small veins that receive blood from the capillaries and deliver it to the larger veins for its return trip to the heart.

Types of veins

In the lower half of the body, where venous ulcers develop, there are three major types of veins:

■ *Superficial veins* lie just beneath the skin and drain into deep veins through perforator veins. Varicose veins are superficial veins that have become stretched and tortuous.

■ *Perforator veins* connect the superficial veins to the deep veins. Their name is derived from the fact that they perforate the deep fasciae as they connect, like rungs on a ladder, superficial veins to the deep venous system.

■ *Deep veins* receive venous blood from the perforator veins and return it to the heart. The major deep veins in the leg include the posterior tibial veins, anterior tibial veins, peroneal veins, and popliteal veins. Each of these veins parallels a corresponding artery. (See *Looking at major leg and foot veins.*)

Vein walls and valves

Compared to arteries of the same size, veins have thinner walls and wider diameters. Vein walls have three distinct layers: an inner, endothelial layer (tunica intima); a middle layer of smooth muscle (tunica media); and an outer, supportive layer (tunica adventitia).

Veins also have a unique system of cup-shaped valves that open toward the heart. The valves keep blood flow-

Looking at major leg and foot veins

Venous ulcers most commonly occur in the legs and feet. This illustration shows the major veins in the lower portion of the body.

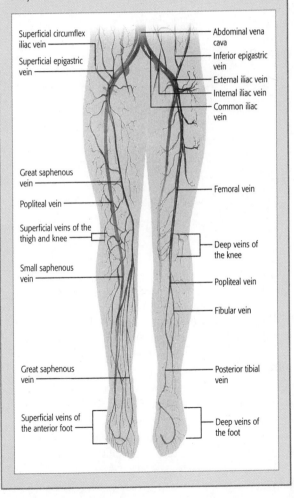

A close look at a vein

This cross section of a vein illustrates the three layers of the vein wall and its unique cup-shaped valves. These valves open toward the heart and, when closed, prevent blood from flowing backward.

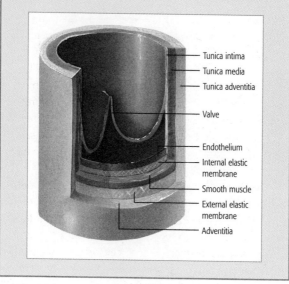

Tunica intima
Tunica media
Tunica adventitia

Valve

Endothelium
Internal elastic membrane
Smooth muscle
External elastic membrane
Adventitia

ing in one direction—toward the heart. Deep veins have more of these valves than superficial veins, and veins in the lower leg have more of these valves than veins in the thigh. In perforator veins, the valves open toward the deep veins. (See *A close look at a vein*.)

Calf muscles have an important role in venous circulation. As calf muscles contract, they squeeze veins in the leg, forcing venous blood toward the heart. When they relax, veins in the leg expand and refill with blood from superficial and perforator veins. This pumping action is important; about 90% of venous blood travels to the heart this way. The other 10% of venous blood empties directly into the vena cava from the great saphenous vein. Calf muscles must be active, however, for the calf muscle pump to work. Leg muscle paralysis or prolonged inactivity eliminates the calf muscle pump and inhibits venous blood flow.

CAUSES

Venous ulcers are the end stage of venous hypertension, which, in turn, results from venous insufficiency. Venous insufficiency simply means that the flow of venous blood from the legs to the heart isn't what it should be. In most cases, incompetent valves are to blame. Valve incompetency may be caused by a thrombus (blood clot) that renders the valve useless or by venous wall distention that separates valve cusps to the point where they no longer meet when the valve closes.

When the flow of venous blood slows, blood pools in the veins of the legs, and venous pressure rises. As the disease progresses, blood backs up through the perforator veins into superficial veins, causing varicose veins to develop in the superficial system. In many cases, edema develops as excess interstitial fluid accumulates. Keep in mind, however, that a patient with varicose veins may not have deep vein insufficiency; vascular tests can differentiate between these two problems.

Venous ulcers can occur in patients with superficial or perforator disease as well as those with deep vein disease. In all cases, however, the underlying problem usually is venous hypertension.

PATIENT CARE

Proper care of venous ulcers includes a thorough knowledge of the patient's history and physical examination.

History

Review the history of the patient's experience with venous ulcers. Note his responses to such questions as:

- When did he first notice this ulcer?
- Is this the first time he has had an ulcer or is this a recurrence?
- If it's a recurrence, what type of treatment did he receive in the past? What type of pain management proved effective?
- Does he have a history of varicose veins? Venous thromboses? Arterial disease? Bleeding problems of any type? Leg trauma? Leg swelling?
- Does he use tobacco?

Physical examination

Record the size of the ulcer (length, width, and depth) and its location. Note necrosis, drainage, or edema. Record the patient's description of pain from the ulcer. Pain may vary from nonexistent to extreme.

Venous ulcers may occur anywhere from the ankle to midcalf; however, they're most common around the middle of the ankle above the malleolus and may extend all the way around the leg. Most have an irregular shape. The borders may have dry crusts or be moist and slightly macerated from drainage. The ulcer itself is shallow with a base of beefy red granulation tissue. The surface may be covered by a yellow film or gray necrotic tissue. Black necrotic tissue is rarely present unless an acute injury has occurred. Check for edema and other signs of venous insufficiency. (See *Identifying venous insufficiency.*)

In venous insufficiency, red blood cells (RBCs), fluid, and fibrin leak into tissues. Note the color of the patient's skin. Hyperpigmentation is common even when ulcers aren't present. This color change is due to a buildup of hemosiderin in the interstitial tissue as the RBCs that have

Identifying venous insufficiency

In a patient with venous insufficiency, check for ulcerations around the ankle. Pulses are present but may be difficult to find if edema is present. The foot may become cyanotic when dependent.

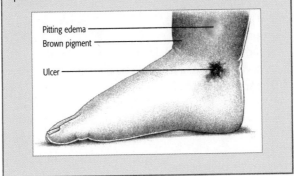

Pitting edema
Brown pigment
Ulcer

leaked into the tissue break down. The fibrin causes skin and subcutaneous tissue to thicken and become fibrotic— a condition called *lipodermatosclerosis*.

Other skin changes characteristic of venous insufficiency include edema, eczema, and atrophie blanche:

■ Edema is one of the first signs of venous disease. It may be confined to the foot or the ankle or may involve the entire leg.

■ Eczema is common, especially in patients who have recurrent ulcers. Skin over scar tissue and edematous tissue is fragile. Drainage from larger ulcers—or medications themselves—can irritate the skin and aggravate eczema.

■ Atrophie blanche may appear as spots of ivory-white plaque in the skin, usually surrounded by hyperpigmentation. Some patients feel discomfort in these areas.

DIAGNOSTIC TESTING
Diagnostic tests for venous ulcers include plethysmography, venous duplex scanning, and venography.

Plethysmography
Plethysmography records changes in the volumes and sizes of extremities by measuring changes in blood volume. There are two types:
- Air plethysmography uses an inflatable pneumatic cuff placed around the limb to obtain volume measurements and standing and walking pressures.
- Photoplethysmography uses infrared light transmitted through the skin to measure venous reflux and filling times. Delayed healing can be predicted by abnormal filling times.

Venous duplex scanning
Venous duplex scanning is used to assess venous patency and reflux by measuring and recording venous pressures along an extremity as its veins are compressed and released. An experienced technician can use venous duplex scanning to identify thrombosis within a vein and determine whether it's acute or chronic as well as to assess venous reflux and the status of valve function. The accuracy of the results depends entirely on the technician's skill.

Venography
Venography is the radiographic examination of a vein injected with a contrast medium. It was once the only test available to evaluate venous thrombosis; however, with the availability of newer, noninvasive tests, venography is now rarely performed.

TREATMENT

Effective treatment of a venous ulcer involves caring for the wound and managing the underlying venous disease. Controlling edema is the most important goal in managing chronic venous insufficiency. Ways to control edema include:

■ elevating the affected leg
■ compression therapy
■ drugs
■ surgery.

Wound care involves selecting the best dressing for a venous ulcer.

Elevating the limb

The most effective method of reducing edema is to elevate the leg and allow gravity to drain the fluid. This is best accomplished with the patient in bed with his legs elevated above the level of his heart. A patient with a cardiac or pulmonary condition may find this position intolerable; in this case, any elevation that the patient can tolerate is beneficial.

Compression therapy

Compression bandages are useful when a patient can't elevate the affected leg. They're also helpful when a patient is on his feet. Various rigid and flexible models are available. Before a compression bandage is added to the treatment regimen, however, ankle brachial index (ABI) should be evaluated to ensure the adequacy of arterial supply.

UNNA BOOT

An *Unna boot*, a commercially prepared, inelastic, medicated gauze compression bandage, is one of the oldest treatments for venous ulcers. It's also one of the most widely used compression bandages because it's inexpensive and effective. This dressing is especially useful for patients who pick at sores because it renders the ulcer inaccessible. The dressing should be changed weekly or more frequently if needed.

An Unna boot consists of a gauze roll that's impregnated with zinc oxide, calamine, and glycerin; it's placed over the skin from below the toes to just below the knee. Any concavity over the ulcer is filled with additional dressing. This dressing is covered with cotton dressings to pad the wound and to absorb drainage. An elastic bandage is wrapped around the outside to provide compression. As the dressing dries, it becomes semirigid. (See *How to wrap an Unna boot.*)

Although an Unna boot provides compression, protection, and a moist environment for healing, its most significant feature is its rigidity. Calf muscle contractions are vital to the effectiveness of an Unna boot. As the patient walks, the rigid dressing restricts outward movement of the calf muscle, directing more of the contraction force inward and improving the function of the calf muscle pump and, in turn, venous circulation. Therefore, an Unna boot is much less effective for a sedentary or bedridden patient. If the patient finds the firmness against the ulcer uncomfortable, place a hydrocolloid or foam dressing over the ulcer before applying an Unna boot.

COMPRESSION STOCKINGS

Compression stockings are essential for long-term management of lower extremity venous disease. They're available in four classes of pressure, as measured at the ankle. Each package of stockings has a list of indications on the label; however, most health care professionals rely on their own experience when choosing a class for a specific patient with a specific problem. Be aware that a patient

SPOTLIGHT

How to wrap an Unna boot

To wrap an Unna boot, follow these steps:
● Clean the patient's skin thoroughly and then flex his knee.
● With the foot positioned at a right angle to the leg, wrap the medicated gauze bandage firmly—not tightly—around the patient's foot. Make sure the dressing covers the heel.
● Continue wrapping upward, overlapping the layers by 50% with each turn. Make sure the dressing circles the leg at an angle to avoid compromising the circulation. Smooth the boot with your free hand as you go, as shown.
● Stop wrapping about 1″ (2.5 cm) below the knee, as shown. If constriction develops as the dressing hardens, make a 2″ (5-cm) slit in the boot just below the knee.
● If drainage is excessive, wrap a roller gauze dressing over the boot.
● Finally, wrap the boot with an elastic bandage in a figure-eight pattern.

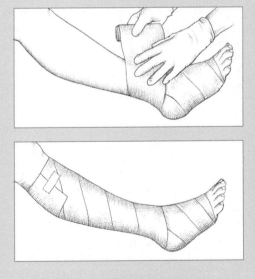

with arthritis, back problems, or obesity may need assistance putting on compression stockings.

CircAid Thera-Boot

If compression stockings or an Unna boot aren't viable options, a CircAid Thera-Boot may be the answer. This dressing provides approximately 30 to 40 mm Hg of compression and is easier to put on than compression stockings, as long as the patient can bend down to reach his legs. The CircAid Thera-Boot is made of a nonelastic semirigid material and has easy-to-use straps that secure the dressing in place. This dressing is washable and reusable and can be removed at night and then put back on in the morning.

Layered compression bandages

Layered compression bandages with three or four layers are relatively new additions to the list of dressing options:

- The first layer is cotton wool, which protects the skin and absorbs moisture. This layer can be pulled apart and repositioned to fill concavities and create a more uniform fit.
- In some versions, the second layer is a support bandage. This layer provides a smooth surface for the compression layers above.
- The next layer is a light compression bandage that provides about 17 mm Hg of pressure.
- The final layer is a compression bandage that provides 23 mm Hg of pressure.

Elastic bandages

Elastic bandages are inexpensive wraps that may be used for compression. They may be short- or long-stretch. (See *Recognizing short-stretch and long-stretch bandages.*)

Recognizing short-stretch and long-stretch bandages

- Short stretch: low working pressure; high resting pressure
- Long stretch: constant, even pressure

A short-stretch bandage has limited elastic stretch, typically less than 90% of its length. When stretched to its limit, a short-stretch bandage becomes semirigid, providing compression while the patient is active. When the patient rests, the dressing provides less compression, protecting the skin from unnecessary pressure. This type of bandage is characterized as providing high working pressure and low resting pressure.

A long-stretch bandage stretches to more than 140% of its length. Long-stretch bandages provide low working pressure and high resting pressure. A long-stretch bandage exerts a specific amount of pressure all the time, whether the patient is active or resting and may provide more pressure than is desirable during periods of rest.

GRADUATED COMPRESSION SUPPORT HOSIERY

Graduated compression support stockings provide a pressure gradient that's greatest at the ankle and lowest at the top of the stocking. This compression is consistent with the hydrostatic pressure in leg veins, which is greatest at the ankle and then diminishes up the leg. These stockings exert 100% of their pressure at the ankle, 70% at the calf, and 40% at the thigh level, producing a pressure gradient that helps reduce venous reflux. Knee-high length stockings are all that's necessary to treat edema from venous hypertension.

Using drugs for venous ulcers

ANTIBIOTICS
Antibiotics may be ordered to treat infection. In most instances, they're given systemically because topical antibiotics aren't effective in treating wound infections; in fact, they may interfere with healing. If the patient is a candidate for skin grafting, topical antibiotics may be used to kill surface bacteria before the procedure.

DIURETICS
Diuretics shouldn't be used to treat edema in cases of venous insufficiency because edema is typically treated in these cases with compression and limb elevation. If the patient has concomitant heart failure, diuretics may be prescribed to treat that condition. Because diuretics can cause volume depletion and serious metabolic disorders, monitor the patient closely.

Compression pumps may be used in conjunction with support hosiery. These devices are available with sleeves that intermittently inflate. They may have a single chamber or separate bladders that inflate sequentially to improve blood flow.

Drugs and surgery

Drugs are rarely prescribed to treat venous ulcers. (See *Using drugs for venous ulcers.*)

Venous ulcers are a chronic disorder. As such, they're slow to heal and recur frequently. Consequently, surgery is rarely a viable treatment. Large surface defects may require repair by skin grafting, but this is a temporary solution. The underlying problem of venous hypertension remains and, in time, edema beneath the scar tissue breaks down the scar and creates another ulcer.

Valve transplant, which involves replacing a section of vein containing a defective valve with a section of vein containing a healthy valve, is performed selectively and almost never for a patient with venous ulcers because by the time an ulcer forms, venous disease is so pervasive that replacing a single valve won't help.

Another surgical procedure called *subfascial endoscopic perforator surgery* (SEPS) may be performed more often. In SEPS, which is based on the theory that incompetent perforator veins cause ulcers at the ankles, faulty perforator veins are located and ligated, redirecting blood flow to healthy veins and improving ulcer healing.

Venous ulcer care

Choosing the proper dressing is an important part of wound care because it affects wound healing. Occlusive dressings are typically selected for venous ulcers because they promote growth of granulation tissue and reepithelialization. If an ulcer contains necrotic debris, a moist gauze dressing or hydrocolloid dressing can be used to provide autolytic debridement. It's appropriate to select a dressing that promotes moist wound healing even though venous ulcers typically produce copious amounts of drainage. Hydrocolloid dressings and some foam dressings retain moisture in the wound while absorbing light to moderate drainage. More absorbent dressings can be used for venous ulcers with moderate to heavy drainage.

Newer therapies can also aid in healing chronic venous ulcers. Preliminary studies show that growth factors can be used to improve the healing rate in venous ulcers. In addition, a bioengineered skin equivalent called *Apligraf* can be used on venous ulcers that fail to heal within 4 weeks of treatment.

Arterial ulcers

Arterial ulcers, which are also called *ischemic ulcers*, are the result of tissue ischemia due to arterial insufficiency. They occur at the distal (farthest) end of an arterial branch and account for 5% to 20% of all leg ulcers.

ARTERIAL ANATOMY AND FUNCTION

Like vein walls, artery walls have three layers:

- The tunica intima, the innermost layer, is a single layer of endothelial cells on a layer of connective tissue.
- The tunica media, the middle layer, is a thick layer of smooth-muscle cells, collagen, and elastic fibers.
- The tunica adventitia, the strong outer layer, is comprised of connective tissue, collagen, and elastic fibers. (See *A close look at an artery.*)

Arteries carry blood leaving the heart to every functioning cell in the body. Their strong, muscular walls allow arteries to expand and relax with each heartbeat, smoothing the powerful pulse to an almost constant pressure by the time blood reaches the capillaries. The lower portion of the body receives its arterial flow through the abdominal aorta and the major arteries that branch from it. (See *Looking at major leg and foot arteries,* page 148.)

CAUSES

Arterial insufficiency occurs when arterial blood flow is interrupted by an obstruction or by narrowing of an artery (arterial stenosis). Occlusion can occur in any artery—from the aorta to a capillary—and can result from trauma or chronic ailment. In time, arterial insufficiency leads to arterial ulcers.

The most common cause of occlusion is atherosclerosis. Patients at highest risk for atherosclerosis include males, cigarette smokers, and individuals with diabetes

A close look at an artery

This cross section of an artery illustrates the layers that comprise the arterial wall.

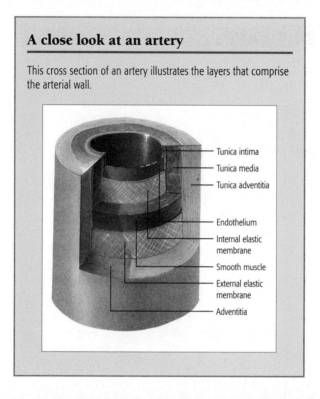

Tunica intima

Tunica media

Tunica adventitia

Endothelium

Internal elastic membrane

Smooth muscle

External elastic membrane

Adventitia

mellitus, hyperlipidemia, or hypertension. Advanced age places patients at even greater risk because, as aging occurs, the tunica intima thickens and loses elasticity. Thickening of the intima is one cause of arterial stenosis.

WARNING SIGNS

In many cases, no signs of arterial insufficiency are apparent until the affected individual suffers an injury. As the demand for additional blood flow to the site of the injury outpaces an occluded artery's ability to deliver it, ischemia occurs. Ischemia is a reduction in the flow of blood to any organ or body part. The primary symptom of ischemia is

Looking at major leg and foot arteries

This illustration identifies the major arteries in the lower portion of the body.

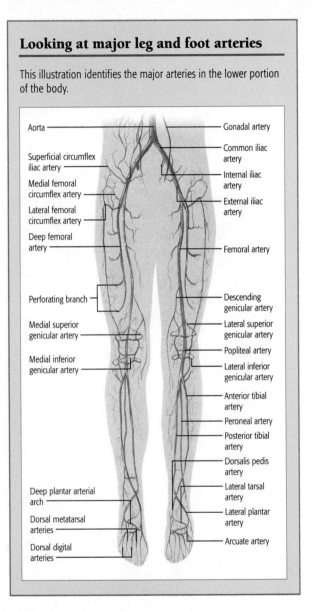

Aorta

Superficial circumflex iliac artery

Medial femoral circumflex artery

Lateral femoral circumflex artery

Deep femoral artery

Perforating branch

Medial superior genicular artery

Medial inferior genicular artery

Deep plantar arterial arch

Dorsal metatarsal arteries

Dorsal digital arteries

Gonadal artery

Common iliac artery

Internal iliac artery

External iliac artery

Femoral artery

Descending genicular artery

Lateral superior genicular artery

Popliteal artery

Lateral inferior genicular artery

Anterior tibial artery

Peroneal artery

Posterior tibial artery

Dorsalis pedis artery

Lateral tarsal artery

Lateral plantar artery

Arcuate artery

pain, which can be severe. This pain may progress from claudication to rest pain.

Claudication

Claudication has been described as "angina of the leg muscles" because the cause of both is an insufficient supply of oxygen. In heart muscle, this deficiency causes the pain of angina. In leg muscles, the same deficiency causes the pain of claudication.

Claudication can occur in any muscle distal to a narrowed artery; it:

■ is brought on by exercise

■ is relieved by rest

■ occurs at a specific distance and is reproducible.

Typically, patients report claudication pain in the calf, thigh, or buttocks. It's measured by how many city blocks (or equivalent distance) the patient can walk before needing to stop to relieve the pain. Factors that tend to shorten the distance traveled before pain occurs include obesity, smoking, and progressive atherosclerotic disease.

Unlike angina, patients experiencing claudication don't have to sit or adopt a particular position to relieve the discomfort; merely stopping reduces the oxygen demand and relieves the pain. As arterial insufficiency progresses, the distance shortens until, ultimately, the patient feels pain even when resting.

Rest pain

Rest pain commonly occurs in the foot and can occur when the patient is asleep. Getting up and walking may provide some relief; however, lowering the extremity provides the most relief. Gravity helps blood flow into the foot and calf, reducing the oxygen deficit and relieving discomfort. By the time rest pain occurs, tissues in the foot are severely ischemic, whether or not an ulcer is present. Unless arterial flow is restored, the patient may face amputation.

PATIENT CARE

Care of arterial ulcers requires a thorough knowledge of the patient's history and physical examination.

History

A patient history reveals whether the patient's wound is an arterial ulcer caused by arterial insufficiency:

▪ If the patient experienced pain and described intermittent claudication, note how far he could walk before pain set in.

▪ If the patient had pain while resting, note when he first noticed it and what measures relieved the pain.

▪ If the patient's pain is in the foot, note if getting up or hanging that foot over the edge of the bed helped. Note which position is most comfortable. Many patients spend their nights sleeping in a chair because the arterial pressure in the leg is too low to perfuse tissues while the leg is extended.

▪ Note smoking history. If the patient smokes, note how long he has been a smoker and how much he smokes.

Physical examination

Inspect the common sites of arterial ulcers: the tips of toes, the corners of nail beds on the toes, over bony prominences, and between toes. The edges of arterial ulcers are well demarcated. Because there's little blood flow to the tissue, the base of the ulcer is pale and dry, and no granulation tissue is present. There may be an area of wet necrosis or a dry scab. The skin surrounding the ulcer feels cooler than normal on palpation. (See *Identifying arterial insufficiency.*)

Identifying arterial insufficiency

Arterial ulcers most commonly occur in the area around the toes. In a patient with arterial insufficiency, the foot usually turns deep red when dependent and the nails may be thick and ridged. In addition, pulses may be faint or absent; the skin is cool, pale, and shiny; and the patient may report pain in his legs and feet.

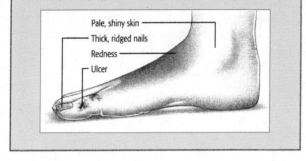

Next, elevate the foot with the ulcer to a 30-degree angle; the skin color in an ischemic foot pales. Ask the patient to place his foot in a dependent position. Ischemic skin becomes deep red as the tissue refills with blood. This dramatic color change is called *dependent rubor*—a sign of severe tissue ischemia. The nails may be thin and pale yellow, or they may have thickened due to an existing fungal infection in the nail beds. A Doppler signal may be heard over small arteries, but this doesn't signify blood flow that's sufficient enough to heal the ulcer.

Palpate the femoral, popliteal, posterior tibial, and dorsalis pedis pulses in each leg and compare your findings with those previously documented. An embolus can occlude an artery and cause ischemia. "Blue toe syndrome," a painful, ischemic toe, is caused by embolic debris in the arteries that supply the toe. (See *Palpating leg and foot pulses,* page 152.)

Palpating leg and foot pulses

These illustrations show where to position your fingers when palpating for pulses of the legs and feet. Use your index and middle fingers to apply pressure.

FEMORAL PULSE
Press relatively hard at a point inferior to the inguinal ligament. For an obese patient, palpate in the crease of the groin, halfway between the pubic bone and the hip bone.

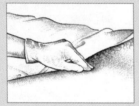

POPLITEAL PULSE
Press firmly in the popliteal fossa at the back of the knee.

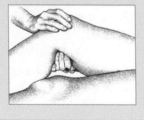

POSTERIOR TIBIAL PULSE
Apply pressure behind and slightly below the middle of the malleolus.

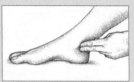

DORSALIS PEDIS PULSE
Place your fingers on the medial dorsum of the foot while the patient points his toes down. The pulse is difficult to palpate here and may seem to be absent in healthy patients.

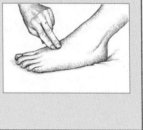

Keep in mind that an absent dorsalis pedis pulse may not be an abnormal finding. Under normal conditions, some patients don't have a palpable dorsalis pedis pulse. Pulses can be palpated when the blood pressure is about 80 mm Hg. If there's no palpable pulse, the blood pressure is probably less than 80 mm Hg. Pulses aren't palpable in a foot with an arterial ulcer.

Compare the color of both legs with each other, and palpate each leg for temperature. A difference in temperature of 10 degrees or more can be noted by palpation. While patient lies down, elevate both of his feet to a 30-degree angle. Watch for a color change. Compress the great toe bilaterally and compare the capillary refill of each side. Normal tissue should refill in less than 3 seconds.

DIAGNOSTIC TESTS

Diagnostic tests commonly used to assess arterial flow to the extremities include segmental pressure recordings, Doppler ultrasonography, ABI, transcutaneous oxygen measurement, and arteriography.

Segmental pressure recordings

Blood pressure is performed to assess the adequacy of arterial blood flow to the legs. Normally, blood pressure readings taken in the arm and the leg should be the same when the patient is lying down. A lower reading in the legs indicates an arterial blockage that may be caused by such problems as a thrombus, cholesterol, or pressure on the outside of the artery.

Blood pressure is measured in both arms while the patient is lying down. Then blood pressure is measured at several points along each leg. Each reading is accompanied by a waveform tracing of the pulse at the time. The entire procedure takes only 20 to 30 minutes. In some cases, the procedure is repeated after a short period of controlled exercise. In arterial insufficiency, arterial blood flow during exercise fails to keep up with the demand of the muscles. Changes in the waveforms and Doppler sig-

How the Doppler probe works

The Doppler ultrasound probe directs high-frequency sound waves through layers of tissue. When the sound waves strike red blood cells (RBCs) moving in the bloodstream, the frequency of the sound waves changes in proportion to the velocity of the RBCs. A recording of these waves facilitates detection of arterial and venous obstruction.

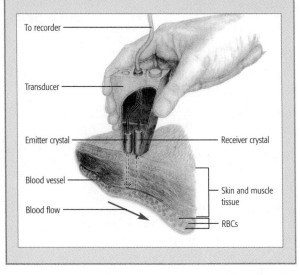

To recorder

Transducer

Emitter crystal

Receiver crystal

Blood vessel

Skin and muscle tissue

Blood flow

RBCs

nals should occur at the same time the patient reports symptoms of claudication.

Doppler ultrasonography

In Doppler ultrasonography, sound waves are used to assess blood flow. This test may be used alone or in conjunction with other diagnostic tests to assess arterial blood flow. During the procedure, a handheld transducer directs high-frequency sound waves into the artery being

Interpreting ABI results

This chart will help you interpret ankle-brachial index (ABI) calculations. Keep in mind that ABI results aren't reliable for patients with diabetes.

ABI	INTERPRETATION
> 0.9	Normal
0.5 to 0.9	Claudication
< 0.5	Resting ischemic pain
< 0.2	Gangrene

tested. Sound waves that strike moving RBCs change frequency—a Doppler shift—in relation to the velocity of the RBCs. The graphic record of these waveforms is then reviewed to determine whether an obstruction exists. (See *How the Doppler probe works.*)

Ankle-brachial index

ABI is a value derived from blood pressure measurements that, taken as a whole, illustrates the progress of arterial disease—or degree of improvement—in the affected limb. Each value in the index is a ratio of a blood pressure measurement in the affected limb to the systolic blood pressure in the brachial arteries. Improvement, or lack thereof, becomes clear when the most recent value is compared to prior values. (See *Interpreting ABI results.*)

The index can also be used to assess treatment methods. Comparing a reading taken before surgery, such as bypass surgery or angioplasty, to a reading taken afterward can indicate the procedure's effectiveness.

When measuring ABI, a Doppler ultrasound and a blood pressure cuff are employed. The steps of the procedure are:

■ First, the patient is placed in a horizontal position so the brachial artery and the dorsalis pedis and posterior tibial arteries are at the same level.

■ Next, brachial blood pressure measurements are taken on both sides. If they differ, the higher of the two systolic pressures is used to calculate the ABI.

■ The blood pressure cuff is wrapped around the ankle just above the malleolus.

■ The dorsalis pedis or posterior tibial artery is identified and the Doppler transducer is held over the artery at a 45-degree angle.

■ The blood pressure cuff is inflated until the Doppler signal is no longer heard; then the cuff is slowly deflated. When the Doppler signal returns, the pressure is recorded. This is the ankle systolic pressure.

■ ABI is calculated by dividing the ankle pressure by the higher of the two brachial systolic pressures.

Transcutaneous oxygen measurement

Some vascular laboratories perform transcutaneous oxygen measurement to assess the perfusion of the microvasculature.

In this test, an electrode is attached to the patient's skin using double-sided tape. Room temperature is kept constant to ensure an accurate reading. The patient is monitored for approximately 20 minutes as the measurement is taken.

A transcutaneous oxygen of approximately 40 mm Hg is generally regarded as the cutoff value associated with inability to heal. However, the accuracy and dependability of this test varies.

Arteriogram

Arteriography is an invasive procedure that's only performed if the patient agrees to undergo a corrective procedure for any problem discovered. It's obtained by inserting a catheter into the arterial system, injecting a
radiopaque contrast medium (a contrast medium that
X-rays can't pass through), and taking an X-ray as the
contrast medium is injected. The resulting image shows
the lumen of the artery and any defect present.

The procedure carries drawbacks and some significant
risks:

■ Several drugs must be stopped for a time before the
procedure.

■ Some patients may be allergic to the contrast medium.

■ Possible complications include injury to the artery that
requires emergency surgery and hematoma that requires drainage.

TREATMENT

The first goal in treatment of an arterial ulcer is to reestab-
lish arterial flow. Without oxygenated blood, the ulcer
won't heal. Options for revascularization include arterial
bypass surgery or angioplasty and stents. In addition, the
ulcer must receive appropriate wound care. In general,
drugs aren't effective when arterial insufficiency has advanced to the point that ulcers are present.

Arterial bypass

Arterial bypass is the most common method of restoring
arterial flow. The type and extent of bypass surgery depends on the disease's stage and location and the patient's
general health. The graft may be autogenous (a vessel tak-
en from the patient) or a synthetic material, typically
Dacron, Gore-Tex, or polytetrafluoroethylene.

Angioplasty and stents

Less invasive interventions, such as angioplasty, are becoming more common for treatment of arterial stenosis. During angioplasty, a catheter with a balloon is inserted into the patient's artery. Using fluoroscopy, the surgeon carefully maneuvers the catheter to the portion of the artery narrowed by plaque and then expands the balloon. The expanding balloon crushes the plaque against the wall of the artery, increasing the lumen diameter.

Stents are small metal structures that can be inserted into an artery after angioplasty to hold the artery open. They were developed to extend the amount of time the artery remains open after angioplasty and, with luck, reduce the need for surgery. Stent placement is still relatively new and the success rate of this procedure has yet to be determined. However, stents may be an alternative for a patient who's considered too high risk for surgery.

Caring for arterial ulcers

Use these procedures when caring for a patient with an arterial ulcer.

■ Keep the arterial ulcer dry and protected from pressure. For a toe ulcer, place small alcohol pads between the toes and change them daily. As the alcohol dries, it promotes a dry ulcer bed. Never soak arterial ulcers. Ischemic tissue macerates in water, increasing the extent of tissue loss, and promoting bacterial growth.

■ Make sure the patient's foot is protected at all times. Consider using a large, bulky dressing or protective footgear—there are many types to choose from. Keep in mind that ischemic tissue can easily develop additional ulcers with little irritation or pressure. Even pressure from the foot resting on the bed or an ill-fitting protective boot can initiate new ulcers. If your patient opts for foot protection, check the device carefully for possible pressure points.

■ If the ulcer area contains necrotic tissue or develops dry gangrene, continue to apply a dry dressing. However, these areas have no sensation and must be protected from injury. If loss of a toe seems imminent, explain this to the patient and let him talk about his feelings. Having a necrotic toe fall off is a shocking and frightening event for most patients, but it's even more devastating when the patient isn't prepared for it.

■ Carefully monitor the line of demarcation between dead and viable tissues. This area is typically painful and is easily infected. Infected ischemic tissue is treated with I.V. antibiotics.

■ If revascularization succeeds, the type of dressing should change. At this point, the wound can be treated according to the rule, "Keep moist tissues moist, and dry tissues dry." Use a dressing that keeps the wound bed moist and the surrounding tissue dry. Consider using a hydrocolloid or hydrogel dressing. Use a moist dressing in the wound bed and cover this with a dry dressing for protection. When securing the dressing, remember to tape from one area of the dressing to another—limit contact with the patient's skin.

Lymphatic ulcers

Lymphatic ulcers, which result from injury in the presence of lymphedema, occur most commonly on the arms and legs. Lymphedema leaves the skin vulnerable to infection and creates skin folds that trap moisture. These conditions cause ulcerations that become difficult to treat.

LYMPHATIC ANATOMY AND FUNCTION

The lymphatic system is a component of the peripheral vascular system. Lymph is a protein-rich fluid similar to plasma. As lymph circulates through lymphatic vessels, it collects wastes, including bacteria, and transports them to lymph nodes. The nodes filter wastes out of the lymph and add lymphocytes to the fluid. Lymph moves slowly through the lymphatic system, driven by muscle contraction and filtration.

CAUSES

Lymphedema is swelling that occurs when an obstruction prevents the normal flow of lymph into venous circulation. Injury to the swollen tissue may cause an ulcer that's slow to heal.

Lymphedema may be congenital or acquired. Acquired lymphedema can be caused by surgery that severs or removes lymph nodes—radical mastectomy, for example—or it may result from compression of a vessel or node due to obesity or unrelated chronic swelling. For instance, patients with chronic venous hypertension and insufficiency may eventually develop lymphedema if venous edema is poorly managed.

Patients with lymphedema are susceptible to skin and soft tissue infections and may require long-term treatment with antibiotics. Prophylactic treatment with antibiotics isn't uncommon because lymphedema causes progressive destruction of lymphatic vessels and nodes which, in turn, slowly increases the patient's risk of infection. Recurrent cellulitis (tissue infection) is common.

In the legs, lymphedema causes a steady seepage of fluids into interstitial tissue. In time, skin and underlying tissues become firm and fibrotic. Thickened tissue presses on the capillaries and occludes blood flow to the skin.

Identifying lymphatic ulcers

- Lymphatic ulcers are most common in the ankle area but may develop at any trauma site.
- Ulcers are shallow and may be oozing, moist, or blistered.
- The surrounding skin is usually firm, fibrotic, and thickened by edema.
- Cellulitis may be present.

The resulting poor circulation makes the leg ulcers that occur with lymphedema extremely difficult to treat.

Leg ulcers on lymphedematous tissue are usually the result of traumatic injury or pressure. However, in extreme cases of lymphedema, the folds of tissue develop deep fissures that trap moisture, causing tissue maceration and the start of a new ulcer. (See *Identifying lymphatic ulcers*.)

TREATMENT

Treatment of lymphatic ulcers has two goals:
- to reduce edema (and maintain the reduction)
- to prevent complications such as infection.

Leg elevation is an important part of therapy for patients with lymphedema. However, in cases of long-standing edema, elevation may be ineffective.

A compression pump is another effective method of reducing edema; however, pump use becomes a lifelong part of managing edema. The pump reduces the volume of fluid in a lymphedematous limb. The pressure should be set low, in the range of 30 to 50 mm Hg. After each compression session, patients must put on compression bandages or another compression garment. Without these, progress gained from the pumping is lost as soon as the patient stands or sits upright.

Comprehensive decongestive therapy is a form of massage that has proven effective for some patients. After each session, the affected limb is wrapped with a short-stretch bandage.

Caring for lymphatic ulcers

Wound care for lymphatic leg ulcers is similar to care for venous ulcers. The primary difference is that the risk of infection is much higher for patients with lymphedema. In lymphedema, choose dressings that can manage large fluid loads while protecting surrounding skin, such as foams or other absorbent dressings.

VASCULAR ULCER CARE WRAP-UP

Keep these tips in mind as you care for a patient with a vascular ulcer:

■ Care must address the underlying disorder or the ulcer won't heal. For instance, with venous ulcers, the underlying venous hypertension must be treated. With arterial ulcers, arterial blood flow must be restored.

■ Vascular disease is pervasive, so look for problems in other areas of the body.

■ Be sure to choose the proper dressing for each ulcer. Remember, dressing choice depends on the characteristics of the ulcer as well as the ulcer type. (See *Types of dressings for vascular ulcers.*)

■ For the most part, the wound care rule of keeping dry tissues dry and moist tissues moist applies to vascular wounds. The one exception is an arterial ulcer, which must be kept dry until the area is revascularized. Then the rule applies here as well.

■ When possible, avoid using tape on the patient's skin. Skin affected by vascular disease is fragile and new ulcers form easily.

SPOTLIGHT

Types of dressings for vascular ulcers

Choosing the best type of dressing for your patient's vascular ulcer depends not only on the ulcer type but also on its condition. This chart lists indications and contraindications for each dressing according to ulcer type.

To use the chart, find the type of ulcer you're trying to dress and then look down the column for indications and contraindications for each dressing type. For example, the chart indicates that an alginate dressing can be used to manage copious drainage in a venous ulcer but isn't indicated for arterial ulcers.

DRESSING	VENOUS ULCERS	ARTERIAL ULCERS	LYMPHATIC ULCERS
Alginates	● Use to manage copious drainage.	● Not indicated.	● Not indicated.
Foam	● Use to protect the ulcer. ● Use for absorption underneath a compression dressing.	● Use to protect the ulcer. ● Use with dry gangrene. ● Use for a moist, revascularized ulcer.	● Use to protect the ulcer. ● Use to absorb drainage.
Gauze	● Use for absorption.	● Use for protection and to allow dry gangrene to maintain its dryness.	● Use for absorption or padding. (Don't allow to dry out on the ulcer.)
Hydrocolloids	● Use to promote granulation. ● Use to manage pain. ● Don't use when copious drainage is present.	● Use for autolytic debridement. ● Use for primary dressing after revascularization. ● Don't use on ischemic tissue.	● Use to protect the skin. ● Use to promote epithelialization. ● Don't use when copious drainage is present. ● Don't use when cellulitis is present.

(continued)

Types of dressings for vascular ulcers (*continued*)

DRESSING	VENOUS ULCERS	ARTERIAL ULCERS	LYMPHATIC ULCERS
Hydrogel	● Don't use when copious drainage is present.	● Use to maintain a moist wound bed. ● Use to debride.	● Use to manage pain. ● Use to debride.
Transparent films	● Not indicated.	● Use only after the ulcer is almost completely healed.	● Use to protect fragile skin. ● Don't use when cellulitis is present.

PATIENT TEACHING

For the most part, the success or failure of treatment is in the patient's hands because he has the primary responsibility for caring for this chronic condition. A motivated patient is more likely to adhere to the treatment regimen—a fact you should keep in mind as you prepare patient-teaching sessions. Patient teaching should provide clear instructions and rationales to encourage active patient participation.

Pass along these tips to your patient to promote vascular ulcer healing and reduce his risk of developing new ulcers:

■ "Look at your skin every day. Use lotion on dry, flaky skin."
■ "Frequent walks aid healing."
■ "Flex your feet up and down (as if you were using the gas pedal in the car) frequently when sitting."
■ "Elevate your legs whenever you sit."

- "Wear shoes that fit well, and always wear socks under shoes."
- "Wear compression stockings."
- "Don't sit or stand for long periods of time."
- "Strive to maintain your target weight."
- "Report all skin injuries to your practitioner."
- "Don't smoke."

7

PRESSURE ULCERS

Pressure ulcers are a serious health problem. Although incidence figures vary widely because of differences in methodology, setting, and subjects, data gathered through 10 years of nationwide studies reveal that 10% to 15% of the general population suffers from chronic pressure ulcers. Prevalence in patients with spinal cord injuries, patients in intensive care units, and nursing home residents is higher.

Pressure ulcers cause suffering and diminish:
- quality of life for the patients
- resources and manpower for the health care industry
- monetary wealth of individuals, health insurers, and government agencies.

The problem is such that many insurers and government agencies now track outcomes to discern whether specific interventions help treat pressure ulcers, and they are encouraging prevention, early intervention, and close monitoring by the health care industry. Because pressure ulcers are chronic conditions—they're hard to heal and tend to recur frequently—prevention and early intervention are critical for more effective management.

Data collected from Outcome and Assessment Information Set (OASIS) forms provide a basis for relating these costs to clinical outcomes. The OASIS-B1 form is currently used by home health care agencies, as mandated by the Centers for Medicare and Medicaid Services.

Better disease management in pressure ulcer cases depends on closer collaboration among government agencies, insurers, and health care professionals. There's heartening evidence that this group effort is developing. All involved are paying closer attention to prevention and the effectiveness of interventions, and they're finding better methods of quantifying and sharing results. In addition, the health care objectives for the nation as a whole reflect a better understanding of the problem's severity. *Healthy People 2010* (a report of the nation's near-term health care goals) includes a goal of reducing by 50% the prevalence of pressure ulcers in nursing home residents.

Causes

Pressure ulcers are chronic wounds resulting from tissue death due to prolonged, irreversible ischemia brought on by compression of soft tissue. Pressure ulcers are the clinical manifestation of localized tissue death caused by lack of blood flow in areas under pressure. Chronic wounds are those that:

▪ fail to heal in a timely manner
▪ resist treatment
▪ tend to recur.

Different tissues have different tolerances for compression. Muscle and fat have comparatively low tolerances for pressure, whereas skin has a somewhat higher tolerance. All cells, regardless of tissue type, depend on blood circulation for the oxygen and nutrients they need. Tissue compression interferes with circulation, reducing or completely cutting off blood flow. The result—ischemia—is that cells fail to receive adequate supplies of oxygen and nutrients. Unless the pressure relents, cells eventually die. By the time inflammation signals impending necrosis on the surface of the skin, it's likely that necrosis has occurred in deeper tissues.

Pressure ulcers are most common in areas where pressure compresses soft tissue over a bony prominence in the body—the tissue is pinched between the outer pressure and the hard underlying surface. Other factors that contribute to the problem include shear, friction, and moisture. Planning effective interventions for prevention and treatment requires a sound understanding of the etiology of pressure ulcers.

PRESSURE

Capillaries are connected to arteries and veins through intermediary vessels called *arterioles* and *venules*. In healthy individuals, capillary filling pressure is about 32 mm Hg where arterioles connect to capillaries and 12 mm Hg where capillaries connect to venules. Therefore, external pressure greater than capillary filling pressure can cause problems. In frail or ill people, capillary filling pressures may be much lower. External pressure that exceeds capillary perfusion pressure compresses blood vessels and causes ischemia in the tissues supplied by those vessels.

If the pressure continues long enough, capillaries collapse and thrombose, toxic metabolic by-products accumulate, and cells in nearby muscle and subcutaneous tissues begin to die. Muscle and fat are less tolerant of interruptions in blood flow than skin. Consequently, by the time signs of impending necrosis appear on the skin, underlying tissue has probably suffered substantial damage. Keep this "tip of the iceberg" effect in mind when assessing the size of a pressure ulcer.

When external pressure exceeds venous capillary refill pressure (about 12 mm Hg), capillaries begin to leak. The resulting edema increases the amount of pressure on blood vessels, further impeding circulation. When interstitial pressure surpasses arterial intravascular pressure, blood is forced into nearby tissues (nonblanchable erythema). Continued capillary occlusion, lack of oxygen and nutrients, and buildup of toxic waste leads to necrosis of muscle, subcutaneous tissue and, ultimately, the dermis and epidermis.

The force associated with any given pressure increases as the amount of body surface exposed to the pressure decreases. For example, the force exerted on the buttocks of a person lying in bed is about 70 mm Hg; however, when the same person sits on a hard surface, the force exerted on the ischial tuberosities can be as much as 300 mm Hg. Consequently, bony prominences are particularly susceptible to pressure ulcers. They aren't the only areas at risk; ulcers can develop on any soft tissue subjected to prolonged pressure. (See *Identifying pressure points,* page 170.)

When blood vessels, muscle, subcutaneous fat, and skin are compressed between a bone and an external surface—a bed or chair, for instance—pressure is exerted on the tissues from both the external surface and the bone. In effect, the external surface produces pressure and the bone produces counterpressure. These opposing forces create a cone-shaped pressure gradient. (See *Understanding the pressure gradient,* page 171.)

Although the pressure affects all tissues between these two points, tissues closest to the bony prominence suffer the greatest damage.

Over time, pressure causes a growing discomfort that prompts a person to change position before tissue ischemia occurs. In ulcer formation, an inverse relationship exists between time and pressure. Typically, low pressure for long periods is far more damaging than high pressure for short periods. For example, a pressure of 70 mm Hg sustained for 2 hours or longer almost always causes irreversible tissue damage, whereas a pressure of 240 mm Hg

Identifying pressure points

Arrows show important pressure points on patients in supine, prone, side-lying, and sitting positions.

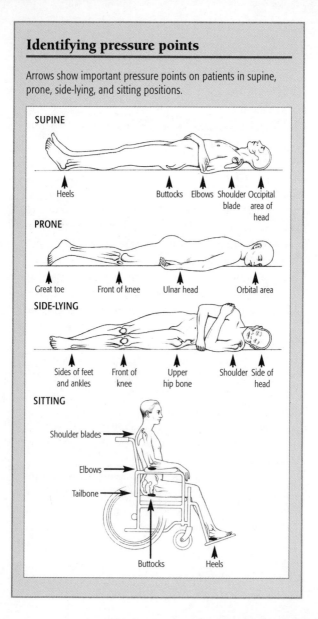

SUPINE

Heels Buttocks Elbows Shoulder blade Occipital area of head

PRONE

Great toe Front of knee Ulnar head Orbital area

SIDE-LYING

Sides of feet and ankles Front of knee Upper hip bone Shoulder Side of head

SITTING

Shoulder blades

Elbows

Tailbone

Buttocks Heels

Understanding the pressure gradient

In this illustration, the V-shaped pressure gradient results from the upward force exerted by the supporting surface and the downward force of the bony prominence. Pressure is greatest on tissues at the apex of the gradient and lessens to the right and left of this point.

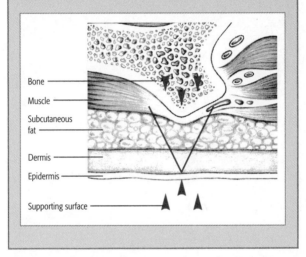

Bone

Muscle

Subcutaneous fat

Dermis

Epidermis

Supporting surface

can be endured for a short time with little or no tissue damage. Furthermore, after the time-pressure threshold for damage passes, damage continues even after the pressure stops. Although pressure ulcers can result from one period of sustained pressure, they're more likely to result from repeated ischemic events without adequate intervening time for recovery.

SHEAR

Shearing force intensifies the pressure's destructive effects. Shear is a mechanical force that runs parallel, rather than

Defining shearing force

Shear is a mechanical force parallel, rather than perpendicular, to an area of tissue. In this illustration, gravity pulls the body down the incline of the bed. The skeleton and attached tissues move, but the skin remains stationary, held in place by friction between the skin and the bed linen. The skeleton and attached tissues actually slide within the skin, causing skin to pucker in the gluteal area.

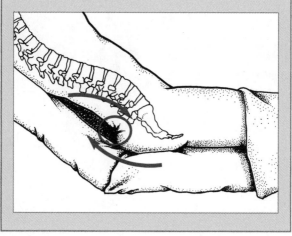

perpendicular, to an area of skin; deep tissues feel the brunt of the force.

Shearing force is most likely to occur during repositioning or when a patient slides down after being placed in high Fowler's position. Simply elevating the head of the bed, however, increases shear and pressure in the sacral and coccygeal areas; gravity pulls the body down but the skin on the back resists the motion because of friction between the skin and the sheets. The result is that the skeleton (and attached tissues) actually slides somewhat beneath the skin (evidenced by the puckering of skin in the gluteal area), generating shearing force between outer layers of tissue and deeper layers. The force generated is enough to obstruct, tear, or stretch blood vessels. (See *Defining shearing force*.)

Shearing force reduces the length of time that tissue can endure a given pressure before ischemia or necrosis occurs. A sufficiently high level of shearing force can cut in half the amount of pressure needed to produce vascular occlusion. Research indicates that shearing force is responsible for the high incidence of triangular shaped, sacral ulcers and the large areas of tunneling or deep undermining beneath these ulcers.

FRICTION

Friction is another potentially damaging mechanical force. Friction develops as one surface moves across another surface—for example, the patient's skin sliding across the bed sheet. Abrasions are wounds created by friction.

Patients at particularly high risk for tissue damage due to friction include those who have uncontrollable movements or spastic conditions, patients who wear braces or appliances that rub against the skin, and older patients. Friction is also a problem for patients who have trouble lifting themselves during repositioning. Rubbing against the sheet can result in an abrasion, which increases the potential for deeper tissue damage. Elevating the head of the bed generates friction between the patient's skin and the bed linen as gravity tugs the patient's body downward. As the skeleton moves inside the skin, friction and shearing force combine to increase the risk of tissue damage in the sacral area. Dry lubricants, such as cornstarch and adherent dressings with slippery backings, can help reduce the impact of friction.

EXCESSIVE MOISTURE

Prolonged exposure to moisture can waterlog, or macerate, skin. Maceration contributes to pressure ulcer formation by softening the connective tissue. Macerated epidermis erodes more easily, degenerates, and eventually sloughs off. In addition, damp skin adheres to bed linen more readily, making friction's effects more profound. Consequently, moist skin is five times more likely to develop ulcers than dry skin. Excessive moisture can result from perspiration, wound drainage, bathing, or fecal or urinary incontinence.

Risk factors

Factors that increase the risk of developing pressure ulcers include advancing age, immobility, incontinence, infection, poor nutrition, and low blood pressure. High-risk patients, whether in a health care facility or at home, should be assessed regularly for pressure ulcers.

AGE

With advancing age, the skin becomes more fragile as epidermal turnover slows, vascularization decreases, and skin layers adhere less securely to one another. Older adults have less lean body mass and less subcutaneous tissue cushioning bony areas. Consequently, they're more likely to suffer tissue damage from friction, shear, and pressure. Other common problems include poor nutrition, poor hydration, and impaired respiratory or immune systems.

IMMOBILITY

Immobility may be the greatest risk factor for pressure ulcer development. The patient's ability to move in response to pressure sensations and the frequency with which his position is changed should always be considered in risk assessment.

INCONTINENCE
Incontinence increases a patient's exposure to moisture and, over time, increases his risk of skin breakdown. Both urinary and fecal incontinence create problems as a result of excessive moisture and chemical irritation. Due to pathogens in the stool, fecal incontinence can cause more skin damage than urinary incontinence.

INFECTION
Although the role of infection in pressure ulceration isn't fully understood, studies in animals on the effects of pressure and infection indicate that compression encourages a localized increase in bacteria concentration. When bacteria was injected into animals, it localized at the compression site and resulted in necrosis at lower pressures relative to the control group. Researchers concluded that compressed skin lowers local resistance to bacterial infection and that infection may reduce the pressure needed to cause tissue necrosis. Furthermore, researchers noted higher infection rates in pedicle flaps when denervation or loss of motor and sensory nerve function occurred. This may explain why neurologically impaired patients are more susceptible to infection and pressure ulceration.

NUTRITION
Proper nutrition is vitally important to tissue integrity. Although a strong correlation exists between poor nutrition and pressure ulceration, nutrition is commonly overlooked during treatment.

Increased protein levels are required for the body to heal itself. Albumin is a key protein in the body. A patient's albumin level is an important indicator of his protein levels. A subnormal albumin level is a late manifestation of protein deficiency. Normal albumin levels range from 3.5 to 5 g/dl. Albumin deficits are classified as:

■ mild: 3 to 3.4 g/dl
■ moderate: 2.7 to 2.9 g/dl
■ severe: less than 2.7 g/dl.

Pressure ulcer occurrence and severity are linked to malnutrition. One recent study found a direct correlation between pressure ulcer stage and degree of hypoalbuminemia (albumin level below 3.5 g/dl). Monitor the albumin levels of a high-risk patient and plan on nutritional intervention if he has hypoproteinemia.

BLOOD PRESSURE

Low arterial blood pressure is clearly linked to tissue ischemia, particularly in patients with vascular impairment. When blood pressure is low, the body shunts blood away from the peripheral vascular system that serves the skin and toward vital organs to ensure their health. As perfusion drops, the skin is less tolerant of sustained external pressure and the risk of damage due to ischemia rises.

Identifying risk factors

Several tools are available to help determine a patient's risk of pressure ulcers. Most are based on the work of Doreen Norton, who studied the pressure ulcer problem in Great Britain. Gosnell and Braden later developed a more refined scale based on data from independent studies. In the last few years, many other researchers have developed assessment tools, giving the clinician many to choose from.

Most tools use these factors to determine a patient's risk of developing pressure ulcers:

■ immobility

- inactivity
- incontinence
- malnutrition
- impaired mental status or sensation.

Each category receives a value based on the patient's condition. The sum of these values determines the patient's score and level of risk. Scores for each category as well as the assessment as a whole help the care team develop appropriate interventions. Most health care facilities require a risk score for every patient admitted. The Agency for Healthcare Quality and Research (AHQR) Guidelines for Pressure Ulcer Prediction and Prevention recommends use of either the Norton or Braden scale.

THE BRADEN SCALE

The Braden scale is the most widely used tool for predicting pressure ulcer risk. This tool scores etiologic factors that contribute to prolonged pressure as well as factors that contribute to diminished tissue tolerance for pressure. Factors scored in this assessment include sensory perception, moisture, activity, mobility, nutrition, and friction and shear. (See *Predicting pressure ulcer risk with the Braden scale,* pages 178 to 181.)

Each factor receives a score of 1 to 4, with the exception of friction and shear, which receives a score of 1 to 3. The highest possible score is 23; the lower the score, the higher the patient's risk of pressure ulceration. A score of 18 or lower denotes a risk of pressure ulcers.

In nursing home populations, most pressure ulcers develop during the first 2 weeks after admission, so early identification of at-risk patients is crucial. No definitive guidelines exist for how often to reassess a patient; however, a common sense approach would be to reassess the patient when his condition changes or if he becomes chair-bound or bedridden.

(Text continues on page 180.)

Predicting pressure ulcer risk with the Braden scale

The Braden scale, shown here, is the most common of several existing tools for determining a patient's risk of developing pressure ulcers. The lower the score, the greater the risk.

SENSORY PERCEPTION Ability to respond meaningfully to pressure-related discomfort	1. Completely limited: Unresponsive (doesn't moan, flinch, or grasp) to painful stimuli because of diminished level of consciousness or sedation OR Limited ability to feel pain over most of body surface	2. Very limited: Responds only to painful stimuli; can't communicate discomfort except by moaning or restlessness OR Has a sensory impairment that limits the ability to feel pain or discomfort over one-half of body
MOISTURE Degree to which skin is exposed to moisture	1. Constantly moist: Skin is kept moist almost constantly by factors such as perspiration and urine; dampness is detected every time patient is moved or turned	2. Very moist: Skin is often but not always moist; linen must be changed at least once per shift
ACTIVITY Degree of physical activity	1. Bedfast: Confined to bed	2. Chairfast: Ability to walk severely limited or nonexistent; can't bear own weight or must be assisted into chair or wheelchair
MOBILITY Ability to change and control body position	1. Completely immobile: Doesn't make even slight changes in body or extremity position without assistance	2. Very limited: Makes occasional slight changes in body or extremity position but can't make frequent or significant changes independently

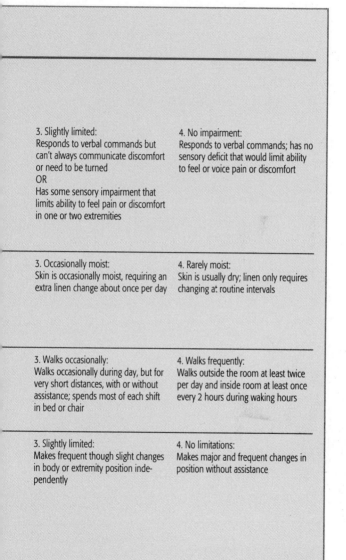

3. Slightly limited:
Responds to verbal commands but can't always communicate discomfort or need to be turned
OR
Has some sensory impairment that limits ability to feel pain or discomfort in one or two extremities

4. No impairment:
Responds to verbal commands; has no sensory deficit that would limit ability to feel or voice pain or discomfort

3. Occasionally moist:
Skin is occasionally moist, requiring an extra linen change about once per day

4. Rarely moist:
Skin is usually dry; linen only requires changing at routine intervals

3. Walks occasionally:
Walks occasionally during day, but for very short distances, with or without assistance; spends most of each shift in bed or chair

4. Walks frequently:
Walks outside the room at least twice per day and inside room at least once every 2 hours during waking hours

3. Slightly limited:
Makes frequent though slight changes in body or extremity position independently

4. No limitations:
Makes major and frequent changes in position without assistance

(continued)

Predicting pressure ulcer risk with the Braden scale *(continued)*

NUTRITION Usual food intake pattern	1. Very poor: Never eats a complete meal; rarely eats more than one-third of any food offered; eats two servings or less of protein (meat or dairy products) per day; takes fluids poorly; doesn't take a liquid dietary supplement OR Is nothing-by mouth status or maintained on clear liquids or I.V. fluids for more than 5 days	2. Probably inadequate: Rarely eats a complete meal and generally eats only about one-half of any food offered; protein intake includes only three servings of meat or dairy products per day; occasionally takes a dietary supplement OR Receives less than optimum amount of liquid diet or tube feeding
FRICTION AND SHEAR	1. Problem: Requires moderate to maximum assistance in moving; complete lifting without sliding against sheets is impossible; frequently slides down in bed or chair, requiring frequent repositioning with maximum assistance; spasticity, contractures, or agitation leads to almost constant friction	2. Potential problem: Moves feebly or requires minimum assistance; during a move, skin probably slides to some extent against sheets, chair restraints, or other devices; maintains relatively good position in chair or bed most of the time but occasionally slides down

Prevention

Pressure ulcer prevention focuses on compensating for prevailing risk factors and addressing the underlying pathophysiology. When planning interventions, be sure to adopt a holistic approach and consider all of the patient's needs.

3. Adequate:
Eats over one-half of most meals; eats four servings of protein (meat, dairy products) each day; occasionally refuses a meal, but usually takes a supplement if offered
OR
Is on a tube feeding or total parenteral nutrition regimen that probably meets most nutritional needs

4. Excellent:
Eats most of every meal and never refuses a meal; usually eats four or more servings of meat and dairy products; occasionally eats between meals; doesn't require supplementation

3. No apparent problem:
Moves in bed and in chair independently and has sufficient muscle strength to lift up completely during move; maintains good position in bed or chair at all times

MANAGING PRESSURE

Managing the intensity and duration of pressure is a fundamental goal in prevention, especially for patients with mobility limitations. Frequent, careful repositioning helps the patient avoid the damaging repetitive pressure that can cause tissue ischemia and subsequent necrosis. When repositioning the patient, it's important to reduce the duration and the intensity of pressure.

Positioning

Each time you reposition the patient, look for telltale areas of reddened skin and make sure the new position doesn't place weight on these areas. Avoid the use of donut-shaped supports or ring cushions that encircle the ischemic area because they can reduce blood flow to an even wider expanse of tissue. If the affected area is on an extremity, use pillows to support the limb or float the heel and reduce pressure. Avoid raising the head of the bed more than 30 degrees to prevent tissue damage due to friction and shearing force.

Inactivity increases a patient's risk of ulcer development. Encourage activity to the degree that the patient is physically able. Start in a small way—help him out of bed and into a chair. As the patient's tolerance improves, help him walk around the room and then down the hall.

Positioning a patient in bed

When the patient is on his side, never allow weight to rest directly on the greater trochanter of the femur. Instead, have the patient rest his weight on his buttock and use a pillow or foam wedge to maintain the position. This position ensures that no pressure is placed on the trochanter or sacrum. A pillow placed between the knees or ankles minimizes the pressure exerted when one limb lies atop the other. (See *Repositioning a reclining patient.*)

Heels present a particularly difficult challenge. Even with the aid of specially designed cushions, reducing the pressure on heels to below capillary refill pressure is almost impossible. Instead, suspend the patient's foot so the bony prominence on the heel is under no pressure. A pillow or foam cushion under the patient's calves can permit a comfortable position while suspending the foot. Take care to avoid knee contraction.

Repositioning a reclining patient

When repositioning a reclining patient, use the Rule of 30—that is, raise the head of the bed 30 degrees (as shown below). Avoid raising the head of the bed more than 30 degrees to prevent the buildup of shearing pressure. When you must raise it more—at meal times, for instance—keep the periods brief.

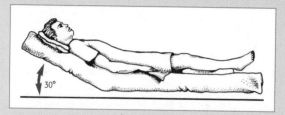

As you reposition the patient from his left side to his right side, make sure his weight rests on his buttock, not his hip bone. This reduces pressure on the trochanter and sacrum. The angle between the bed and an imaginary lateral line through his hips should be about 30 degrees. If needed, use pillows or a foam wedge to help the patient maintain the proper position (as shown below). Cushion pressure points, such as the knees or shoulders, with pillows as well.

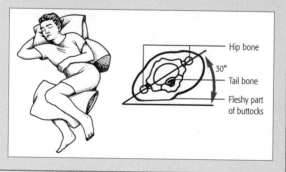

POSITIONING A SEATED PATIENT

As unlikely as it seems, a patient is more likely to develop pressure ulcers from sitting than from reclining. Sitting tends to focus all of the patient's weight on the relatively small surface areas of the buttocks, thighs, and soles. Much of this weight is focused on the small area of tissue covering the ischial tuberosities. Proper posture and alignment help ensure that the weight of the patient's body is distributed as evenly as possible.

Proper posture alone can significantly reduce the patient's risk of ulcers at the ankles, elbows, forearms, wrists, and knees. Explain proper posture to your patient, if necessary, as described here:

■ Have the patient sit with his back erect and against the back of the chair, thighs parallel to the floor, knees comfortably parted, and arms horizontal and supported by the arms of the chair. This posture distributes weight evenly over the available body surface area.

■ Feet should be kept flat on the floor to protect the heels from focused pressure and distribute the weight of the legs over the largest available surface area—the soles.

■ Don't allow the patient to slouch, which causes shearing force and friction and places undue pressure on the sacrum and coccyx.

■ Keep the thighs and arms parallel to ensure that weight is evenly distributed all along the thighs and forearms, instead of being focused on the ischial tuberosities and elbows, respectively.

■ Part the knees to keep knees and ankles from rubbing together.

If the patient uses an ottoman or footstool, determine whether his knees are above the level of his hips. If so, then his weight has shifted from the back of his thighs to the ischial tuberosities—and he needs a different footstool. The same problem—knees above hips—can occur if the chair itself is too short for the patient.

Patients at risk should reposition themselves every 15 minutes while sitting, if they can. Patients with spinal cord injuries can perform wheelchair pushups to intermittently relieve pressure on the buttocks and sacrum. This requires a fair amount of upper body strength, however, and some patients might not have the strength. Others may have injuries that preclude using this technique.

Support aids and cushions

Although pillows may be the most common support tools, they aren't the only options available. There's a vast array of support surfaces and cushioning aids to choose from. Special beds, mattresses, and seating options that employ foams, gels, water, and air as cushioning agents make it possible to tailor a comprehensive and personal system of supports for your patient.

Effective care depends on knowledge of the classes and types of products. In the course of your work, take time to learn as much as you can about these products. (See *Types of devices for reducing pressure,* page 186.)

Be informed, but also be cautious. Using these devices can instill a false sense of security. Remember that as helpful as these devices may be, they aren't substitutes for attentive care. Patients require individual turning schedules regardless of the equipment used.

Beds and mattresses

When we discuss horizontal support surfaces we are, for the most part, talking about beds, mattresses, and mattress overlays. These products employ foams, gels, water, and air to minimize the pressure a patient experiences while lying in bed.

Types of devices for reducing pressure

Special pads, mattresses, and beds are available to help relieve pressure when a patient is confined to one position for long periods. Choices include:

GEL PADS
Gel pads disperse pressure over a wide surface area.

WATER MATTRESS OR PADS
A wave effect provides even distribution of body weight.

ALTERNATING-PRESSURE AIR MATTRESS
Alternating deflation and inflation of mattress tubes changes areas of pressure.

FOAM MATTRESS OR PADS
Foam areas, which must be at least 3″ to 4″ (7.5- to 10-cm) thick, cushion skin and minimize pressure.

LOW-AIR-LOSS BEDS
This bed surface consists of inflated air cushions. Each section is adjusted for optimal pressure relief for the patient's body size.

AIR-FLUIDIZED BED
An air-fluidized bed contains beads that move under an air-flow to support the patient, thus reducing shearing force and friction.

STRYKER OR FOSTER FRAME OR CIRCOLECTRIC BED
These devices relieve pressure by turning the patient.

MECHANICAL LIFTING DEVICES
Lift sheets and other mechanical lifting devices prevent shearing by lifting the patient rather than dragging him across the bed.

PADDING
Pillows, towels, and soft blankets, when properly positioned, can reduce pressure in body hollows.

FOOT CRADLE
A foot cradle lifts the bed linens to relieve pressure over the feet.

BEDS

Specialty beds, such as oscillating and rotating beds, relieve pressure by rotating the patient or helping to lift the patient to reduce the risk of friction and shear. However, they're expensive and are rarely an option for a patient returning home from a health care facility. Remember that no bed takes the place of a patient being turned or repositioned by a health care practitioner.

MATTRESSES

Most mattresses worth considering use some form or manipulation of foam, gel, air, or water to cushion the patient. Foam core mattresses can provide the same benefits derived from a standard mattress with a foam overlay. Low-air-loss and high-air-loss mattresses are specialized support devices that pass air over the patient's skin. These mattresses promote moisture evaporation and are especially useful when skin maceration is a problem. Be alert for signs and symptoms of dehydration in the patient who uses a high-air-loss mattress.

Water mattresses and some air mattresses use different media, but similar techniques, to evenly distribute pressure under the patient. Water mattresses use gentle wave motion to maintain even distribution of pressure, whereas several types of air mattress alternately inflate and deflate tubes within the mattress to distribute pressure.

MATTRESS OVERLAYS

The most common mattress overlays used in pressure ulcer prevention are foam, air, and gel overlays. Foam overlays should be at least 3″ (7.5 cm) thick for the average patient; thicker is even better. Although 2″ (5 cm) foam overlays may add comfort, they aren't suitable for patients at risk for pressure ulcers. Three-inch solid foam is preferable to the convoluted type. Be sure to select an overlay

Testing a foam overlay's effectiveness

To ensure the overlay is effective, hand check whenever a new overlay is put into service or if you suspect an overlay is breaking down. To hand check an overlay, slide one hand—palm up and fingers outstretched—between the mattress overlay and the mattress. If you can feel the patient's body through the overlay, replace the overlay with a thicker one or add more air to the mattress. Another way to evaluate whether a foam overlay has the appropriate denseness is to squeeze the foam between your fingers. If you are able to squish the foam until your fingers touch, the foam won't adequately support the patient's weight.

constructed from higher-quality foam because it will last longer.

If the patient's weight completely compresses a mattress overlay, the overlay won't be effective. (See *Testing a foam overlay's effectiveness.*)

Support aids for sitting

Products designed to help prevent pressure ulcers while sitting fall into two broad categories: products that relieve pressure and products that ease repositioning.

Ambulatory and wheelchair-dependent patients should use seat cushions to distribute weight over the largest possible surface area. Wheelchair-dependent patients require an especially rugged seat cushion that can stand up to the rigors of daily use. In many instances, a good foam cushion 3″ to 4″ (7.5 to 10 cm) thick suffices. However, many wheelchair-seating clinics now use computers to create custom seating systems tailored to fit the physiology and needs of each patient. For patients with spinal cord injuries, the selection of wheelchair seating is based on pressure evaluation, lifestyle, postural stability, continence, and cost. Custom seats and cushions are more expensive; however, in this case, the added expense is justifiable. Encourage wheelchair patients to replace seat cushions as soon as their current one begins to deteriorate.

Repositioning is just as important when the patient is sitting as when he's reclining. For a patient requiring assistance, devices such as overhead frames, trapezes, walkers, and canes can help the patient reposition himself as necessary. Health care personnel can help maneuver I.V. poles and other support equipment.

MANAGING SKIN INTEGRITY

An effective skin integrity management plan includes regular inspections for tissue breakdown, routine cleaning and moisturizing, and steps to protect the skin from incontinence, as appropriate.

Inspecting the skin

The patient's skin should be routinely inspected for pressure areas, depending on his assessed risk and ability to tolerate pressure. Check for pallor and areas of redness—both signs of ischemia. Be aware that redness that occurs after the pressure is removed (called *reactive hyperemia*) is commonly the first external sign of ischemia due to pressure.

Cleaning the skin

Usually, cleaning with a gentle soap and warm water suffices for daily skin hygiene. Use a soft cloth to pat, rather than rub, the skin dry. Avoid scrubbing or the use of harsh cleaning agents.

Moisturizing the skin

Skin becomes dry, flaky, and less pliable when it loses moisture. Dry skin is more susceptible to ulceration. There are numerous skin moisturizing products available; it shouldn't be hard to find one that the patient likes. The three categories of skin moisturizers are lotions, creams, and ointments:

▪ *Lotions* are dissolved powder crystals held in suspension by surfactants. They have the highest water content and evaporate faster than other types of moisturizers. Consequently, lotions must be applied more often. The high water content is the reason lotions feel cool as they're applied.

▪ *Creams* are preparations of oil and water; they're more occlusive than lotions. Creams don't have to be applied as often as lotions; three or four applications per day should be adequate. Creams are better for preventing moisture loss due to evaporation than for replenishing skin moisture.

▪ *Ointments* are preparations of water in oil (typically lanolin or petrolatum). They're the most occlusive and longest lasting form of moisturizer. Studies indicate that petrolatum is a more effective moisturizer than lanolin.

Protecting the skin

Although some moisture is good, too much is a problem. Waterlogged skin is easily eroded by friction and is more susceptible to irritants and bacterial colonization than dry skin. Close monitoring helps head off problems before they escalate.

Skin protection is particularly important if the patient is incontinent. Urine and feces introduce chemical irritants and bacteria as well as moisture, which can speed skin breakdown. To effectively manage incontinence, first determine the cause and then plan interventions that protect skin integrity while addressing the underlying problem.

In older adults, don't assume that incontinence is a normal part of aging. In most cases, factors that influence, increase, or precipitate incontinence are reversible, such as:

■ fecal impaction and tube feeding (can cause diarrhea)
■ a reaction to medication (can cause urinary incontinence or diarrhea)
■ urinary tract infection
■ mobility problems (can keep the patient from reaching the bathroom in time)
■ clothing barriers that make it difficult for the patient to get out of the clothing in time to get to the toilet without soiling himself
■ confusion or embarrassment (can keep the patient from asking for a bedpan or help getting to the bathroom).

Whether the underlying cause is reversible or not, encourage the patient to ask for help when he needs a bedpan or needs to go to the bathroom. Use incontinence collectors, diapers or underpads, and skin barriers as appropriate to minimize skin damage. (See *Managing incontinence*, pages 192 and 193.)

Increase the frequency of inspections, cleansing, toileting, and moisturizing for these patients.

MANAGING NUTRITION

Proper nutrition is essential to both ulcer prevention and healing.

Dietary intake

Protein is particularly important to skin maintenance. Your patient needs a balanced diet that includes about 0.8 g/kg/day of protein. For most healthy adults, this

Managing incontinence

Incontinent patients require careful monitoring and special interventions to prevent skin damage caused by excessive moisture, chemical irritation, or microbial infection. Three types of aids can help you manage incontinence and minimize its impact on your patient: incontinence collectors, incontinence diapers and underpads, and topical barriers.

INCONTINENCE COLLECTORS

● Condom catheters can help manage urinary incontinence in men (similar but less effective devices exist for women).

● Fecal incontinence collectors are pectin skin barriers with an attached, drainable pouch (similar to colostomy pouching systems).

● Fecal collectors need to be changed on a regular schedule and when leakage is noted. Rectal tubes aren't a good alternative because they can cause such complications as vasovagal response or ischemia of anal tissue.

INCONTINENCE DIAPERS AND UNDERPADS

● Diapers and underpads wick moisture away from the patient's skin. Underpads and diaper alternatives include disposable absorbent gel diapers, disposable cellulose core diapers, and laundered reusable cloth diapers.

● Studies indicate that disposable gel diapers are significantly more effective in reducing wetness and maintaining normal skin pH than other alternatives. Reusable cloth diapers offer the least expensive alternative.

● Don't be tempted to put a plastic or paper linen saver under an incontinent patient; this holds moisture next to the patient's skin and compounds the problem.

● Don't secure the pad to the patient. Underpads work by absorbing wetness and allowing air to circulate over the skin, drying it.

● Diapers and underpads require routine monitoring so they can be changed promptly after episodes of incontinence.

TOPICAL SKIN BARRIERS

● Liquid copolymer film barriers protect intact skin from the damaging effects of incontinence. They're available in

Managing incontinence (*continued*)

aerosol form or as disposable wipes. As these products dry, a strong, almost plasticlike barrier forms on the skin's surface that isn't easily washed off during normal cleaning.

● Paste is an excellent skin barrier. A paste is an ointment that contains powder for thickness and durability. Many pastes contain zinc oxide. Pastes can be removed with mineral oil.

means eating one or two 3-ounce servings of protein each day in the form of meat, milk, cheese, or eggs.

Body weight

Low body weight is a problem for many pressure ulcer patients. An underlying illness or anorexia can make eating undesirable or impossible. To prevent problems and to monitor the results of nutritional interventions, weigh the patient weekly. If the patient history includes an unintentional weight loss of 10 lb (4.5 kg) or more during the previous 6 months, malnutrition may be the cause.

Identifying pressure ulcers

Pressure ulcers can occur even with the best preventive measures. Effective treatment depends on a thorough evaluation of the developing wound. Meaningful ulcer care requires a systematic and objective approach. Clinical knowledge of pressure ulcers should include:

■ ulcer history, including etiology, duration, and prior treatment
■ anatomic location

- stage
- size (length, width, depth in centimeters)
- sinus tracts, undermining, and tunneling
- drainage (amount and description, including odor)
- necrotic tissue (slough and eschar and amount)
- granulation tissue (present or not and amount)
- epithelialization (present or not and amount).

Ulcer borders can provide clues to healing potential. Check the skin around the ulcer for:

- redness
- warmth
- induration or hardness
- swelling
- wound edges (open or closed)
- signs of infection.

Before you examine the ulcer, assess the patient's pain. In most cases, pressure ulcers cause some degree of pain; in some cases, pain is severe. Have the patient rate his pain on a visual analog scale of 0 to 10, with 0 representing no pain and 10 representing severe pain. Similarly, ask the patient whether the pain interferes with his ability to function normally and, if so, to what degree.

LOCATION

Ulcers are more common on the lower half of the body because it has more major bony prominences and more body weight than the upper half of the body. Two-thirds of pressure ulcers occur within the pelvic girdle. (See *Identifying common locations for pressure ulcers.*)

CHARACTERISTICS

Tissue involvement ranges from blanchable erythema to the deep destruction of tissue associated with a full-thickness wound. Pressure against tissue interrupts blood flow and causes pallor due to tissue ischemia. If pro-

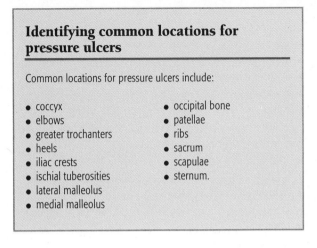

Identifying common locations for pressure ulcers

Common locations for pressure ulcers include:

- coccyx
- elbows
- greater trochanters
- heels
- iliac crests
- ischial tuberosities
- lateral malleolus
- medial malleolus
- occipital bone
- patellae
- ribs
- sacrum
- scapulae
- sternum.

longed, ischemia causes irreversible and extensive tissue damage.

Reactive hyperemia

Usually, reactive hyperemia is the first visible sign of ischemia. When the pressure causing ischemia is released, skin flushes red as blood rushes back into the tissue. This reddening is called *reactive hyperemia*. It's due to a protective mechanism in the body that dilates vessels in the affected area to increase the blood flow and speed oxygen to starved tissues. Reactive hyperemia first appears as a bright flush that lasts about one-half or three-fourths as long as the ischemic period. If the applied pressure is too high for too long, reactive hyperemia fails to meet the demand for blood and tissue damage occurs.

Blanchable erythema

Blanchable erythema (redness) can signal imminent tissue damage. Erythema results from capillary dilation near the skin's surface. In the patient with pressure ulcers, the redness results from the release of ischemia-causing pressure. Blanchable erythema is redness that blanches—turns white—when pressed with a fingertip and then immediately turns red again when pressure is removed. Tissue exhibiting blanchable erythema usually resumes its normal color within 24 hours and suffers no long-term damage. However, the longer it takes for tissue to recover from finger pressure, the higher the patient's risk of developing pressure ulcers.

In dark-skinned patients, erythema is hard to discern. Use bright light and look for taut, shiny patches of skin with a purplish tinge. Also, assess carefully for localized heat, induration, or edema, which can be better indicators of ischemia than erythema.

Nonblanchable erythema

Nonblanchable erythema can be the first sign of tissue destruction. In high-risk patients, nonblanchable tissue can develop in as little as 2 hours. The redness associated with nonblanchable erythema is more intense and doesn't change when compressed with a finger. If recognized and treated early, nonblanchable erythema is reversible.

In many cases, the full extent of ulceration can't be determined by visual inspection because there may be extensive undermining along fascial planes. For example, tunneling can connect ulcers over the sacrum to ulcers over the trochanter of the femur or the ischial tuberosities. These cavities can contain extensive necrotic tissue.

SIZE

Using a disposable measuring tape, measure wound length (in centimeters) as the longest dimension of the wound and width as the longest distance perpendicular to the length. Use the face of a clock as a reference to document where the wound was measured. This will help everyone measure the wound in the same place. Alternatively, carefully trace the wound margins on a piece of paper. In addition, a growing number of facilities use wound photography. Measure the ulcer's depth at its deepest point by inserting a gloved finger or a cotton-tipped swab. If you're using a probe other than your finger, be very careful; it's easy to cause further damage. Note visible tunnels or undermining; if possible, use a gloved finger or sterile cotton swab to gauge the extent.

BASE
The type of tissue in the ulcer base determines the potential for healing and the type of treatment. Know how to identify necrotic tissue, fibrin slough, granulation tissue, and epithelial tissue.

Necrotic tissue
Necrotic tissue may appear as a moist yellow or gray area of tissue that's separating from viable tissue. When dry, necrotic tissue appears as thick, hard, and leathery black eschar. Areas of necrotic or devitalized tissue may mask underlying abscesses and collections of fluid. Before the ulcer can begin to heal, necrotic tissue, drainage, and metabolic wastes must be removed from the wound.

Fibrin slough
Fibrin slough is stringy tissue that is adhered to the wound bed, and may be yellow, tan, gray, or black.

Granulation tissue
Granulation tissue appears as beefy red, bumpy, shiny tissue in the base of the ulcer. As it heals, a full-thickness ulcer develops more and more granulation tissue. Such factors as tissue oxygenation, tissue hydration, and nutrition can alter the color and quality of granulation tissue.

Describing wound drainage

Here are some common descriptive terms for wound drainage
and their meaning to aid you in your documentation:
- serous—clear, watery
- sanguineous—red
- serosanguineous—clear with red or reddish brown
- purulent—thick, yellow, cloudy.

Epithelial tissue

Epithelialization is the regeneration of epidermis across
the ulcer surface. It appears as pale or dark pink skin, first
becoming evident at ulcer borders in full-thickness
wounds and as islands around hair follicles in partial-
thickness wounds. Wound healing can be assessed and
quantified by the percentage of surface covered by new
epithelium.

DRAINAGE

Ulcers with drainage, or exudate, take longer to heal.
Drainage characteristics include amount, color, consistency, and odor. Record the amount as scant, moderate, large,
or copious. Describe the color and consistency together
with clear, descriptive terms. (See *Describing wound drainage*.)

Odor is a subjective observation—one that can suggest infection. It's important to clean the wound thoroughly before assessing the color and odor of drainage.
Otherwise, perceived drainage may be, in actuality, a combination of dressing residue and dead cells—a combination that always produces a noxious odor. However, pu-
trid odor that remains after wound cleaning may indicate
anaerobic infection.

MARGINS

Pressure ulcer edges have distinct characteristics, including color, thickness, and degree of attachment to the wound base.

Assess the epithelial rim as an integral part of the wound base. Ideally, there should be a free border of epithelial cells. These are the cells that proliferate and migrate across the wound bed during healing. When epidermis at the ulcer edges thickens and rolls under, it impairs migration of epithelial cells. In *epiboly*, the wound edges thicken and the pressure ulcer becomes chronic, with little or no evidence of new tissue growth.

In *undermining*, which occurs when necrosis of subcutaneous fat or muscle occurs, a pocket extends beneath the skin at the ulcer's edge. *Tunneling* differs from undermining in that both ends of a tunnel emerge through the skin's surface. In many cases, a tunnel connects two otherwise distinct pressure ulcers; it may be necessary to open the tunnel before the ulcer can heal. To determine whether the patient has undermining or tunneling, remember that in undermining you'll be able to move the cotton-tipped applicator in all directions, whereas in tunneling the cotton-tipped applicator will only go in a line.

Sometimes full-thickness pressure ulcers form tracts along fascial planes. When these are extensive, external palpation is the only way to determine the direction and length of the tracts. If this is necessary, use a felt-tipped pen to outline the tract on the skin and measure the resulting image.

SURROUNDING SKIN

Check intact skin surrounding the ulcer for redness, warmth, induration (hardness), swelling, and signs of infection. Palpate for heat, pain, and edema. The ulcer bed should be moist, but the surrounding skin should be dry.

The skin should be adequately moisturized but neither macerated nor eroded. Macerated skin appears water-logged and may turn white at the wound's edges.

A saline-soaked dressing can cause maceration of surrounding skin, unless the skin is protected. Other common causes of maceration include wound drainage and urine or feces contamination. Irritation or stripping may be the result of poor technique during dressing changes.

Pressure ulcer staging

The most widely used system for staging pressure ulcers is the classification system developed by the National Pressure Ulcer Advisory Panel (NPUAP). This staging system, which defines four stages, has been adopted by the AHQR Pressure Ulcer Guideline Panels and is published in both sets of *AHQR Clinical Practice Guidelines for Pressure Ulcers*. NPUAP is considering rewording the staging system used and adding stages to address gaps in the current wording.

Staging reflects the depth and extent of tissue involvement. Restaging isn't needed unless deeper layers of tissue are exposed by treatments such as debridement. Although staging is useful for classifying pressure ulcers, it's only one part of a comprehensive assessment. Also, if necrotic tissue is covering the wound base, you won't be able to accurately stage the wound. Ulcer characteristics and the condition of the surrounding skin provide equally important clues to the ulcer's prognosis. (See *Staging pressure ulcers*.)

Pressure ulcers can't be back-staged or reversed as they heal. After the subcutaneous tissue, muscle, or bone tissue is damaged or lost, it's replaced by scar tissue, not tissue of the same cellular makeup of the tissue that was lost.

Staging pressure ulcers

When performing pressure ulcer care, evaluate the ulcer for staging, as described here. Staging reflects the anatomic depth of exposed tissue. Keep in mind that if the wound contains necrotic tissue, you won't be able to determine the stage until you can see the wound base.

STAGE I
The first sign of a pressure ulcer is a reddened area of intact skin that doesn't blanch. In a patient with dark skin, the area may be warm, hard, edematous, indurated, and discolored.

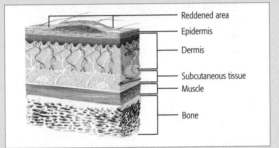

Reddened area
Epidermis
Dermis
Subcutaneous tissue
Muscle
Bone

STAGE II
A stage II ulcer will show partial-thickness skin loss involving the epidermis, the dermis, or both. These superficial ulcers may consist of an abrasion, a blister, or a shallow crater.

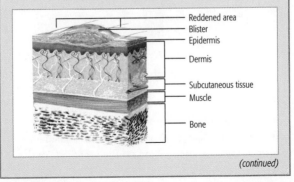

Reddened area
Blister
Epidermis
Dermis
Subcutaneous tissue
Muscle
Bone

(continued)

Staging pressure ulcers *(continued)*

STAGE III
A stage III ulcer is a full-thickness crater-like wound that may extend to underlying fasciae and undermine the connective tissue.

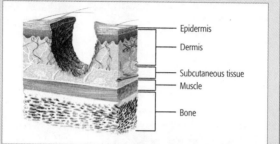

- Epidermis
- Dermis
- Subcutaneous tissue
- Muscle
- Bone

STAGE IV
In stage IV, the wound extends through the skin, damaging muscle, bone, and supporting structures; causing necrosis of tissues; and resulting in undermining and sinus tracts.

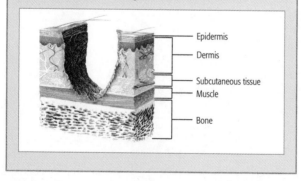

- Epidermis
- Dermis
- Subcutaneous tissue
- Muscle
- Bone

STAGE I

A stage I pressure ulcer is an area of skin with observable pressure-related changes when compared with an adjacent area or to the same region on the other side of the body. Indicators include a change in one or more of these characteristics:

- skin temperature (warmth or coolness)
- tissue consistency (boggy or firm)
- sensation (pain or itching).

This ulcer presents clinically as a defined area of persistent redness (nonblanchable) in patients with light skin or persistent red, blue, or purple in patients with darker skin.

STAGE II
A stage II pressure ulcer is a superficial partial-thickness wound that presents clinically as an abrasion, a blister, or a shallow crater involving the epidermis and dermis. This stage doesn't involve subcutaneous tissue.

STAGE III
A stage III pressure ulcer is a full-thickness wound with tissue damage or necrosis of subcutaneous tissue that can extend down to, but not through, underlying fasciae. The ulcer presents clinically as a deep crater with or without undermining of adjacent tissue.

STAGE IV
A stage IV ulcer involves full-thickness skin loss with extensive damage, destruction, or necrosis to muscle, bone, and supporting structures (such as tendons and joint capsule). Undermining and sinus tracts may also be present.

Closed pressure ulcers

Although the pathology is the same, closed pressure ulcers are unique and potentially life-threatening pressure ulcers. They begin when shearing force causes ischemic necrosis in subcutaneous tissue. No surface defect marks this event. In time, pressure from inflammation in the cavity of necrotic debris causes a small, unremarkable ulcer to form on the skin. This ulcer drains a large contaminated base. There are no signs of systemic infection.

Closed pressure ulcers can't be classified by stage or grade because it's impossible to determine the extent of damage until the defect is surgically opened. In addition, surgery is the preferred treatment.

Patients confined to wheelchairs because of spinal cord injury are at highest risk for this type of pressure ulcer, and the ulcers occur most commonly in the pelvic region. Prompt recognition is crucial. The most viable treatment is wide surgical excision and closure with a muscle rotation flap.

Treatment

Treatment of pressure ulcers follows the four basic steps common to all wound care:
■ Debride necrotic tissue and clean the wound to remove debris.
■ Provide a moist wound-healing environment through the use of proper dressings.
■ Protect the wound from further injury.
■ Provide nutrition essential to wound healing.

A key element in all pressure ulcer treatment plans is identifying and treating, when possible, the underlying pathophysiology. If the cause of the ulcer remains, existing ulcers don't heal or will reopen and new ulcers develop.

Typically, wound care involves cleaning the wound, debriding necrotic tissue, and applying a dressing that keeps the wound bed moist. Topical agents are used to resolve various issues.

WOUND CLEANING

Wound cleaning removes wound debris, old dressing materials, and necrotic tissue from the wound surface. Pressurized wound irrigation is adequate for almost all wound cleaning. (For more information on wound cleaning, see chapter 4, Basic wound care procedures.)

DEBRIDEMENT

Debridement removes nonviable tissue and is the most important factor in wound management. Healing can't take place until necrotic tissue is removed. (For more information on debridement, see chapter 4, Basic wound care procedures.)

DRESSINGS

Dressings serve to:
■ protect the wound from contamination
■ prevent trauma
■ provide compression (if bleeding or swelling occurs)
■ apply medications
■ absorb drainage or debride necrotic tissue.

When choosing a dressing for a pressure ulcer, the cardinal rule remains the same: Keep moist tissue moist and dry tissue dry. Wound characteristics dictate the type of dressing used. The dressing selected should protect wound integrity and keep the wound surface moist but prevent an excessive buildup of moisture, which can cause maceration and bacterial colonization. The frequency of dressing changes depends on the amount and type of wound drainage as well as the characteristics of the dressing.

Wound cavities may require light packing or fill to prevent areas from walling off and developing into abscesses. Be careful with packing, however; too much packing can generate more pressure and cause additional tissue damage.

Patient education

The goal of patient education is to improve the outcome. For a care plan to succeed after the patient leaves the hospital, the patient or caregiver must understand the plan, be physically capable of carrying it out at home, and value both the information and the outcomes. Therefore, education and goal establishment should take into consideration the preferences and lifestyles of the patient and his family whenever possible.

Teach the patient and family members how to prevent pressure ulcers and what to do when they occur. (See *Pressure ulcer do's and don'ts.*)

Explain repositioning, and show what a 30-degree laterally inclined position looks like. If the patient needs assistance with repositioning, make sure he knows the types of devices available and where to obtain them.

Show the patient how he can inspect his back and other areas using a mirror. If the patient can't do this, a family member can help. Make sure he understands the importance of inspecting skin over bony prominences for pressure-related damage every day.

If the patient needs to apply dressings at home, make sure he knows the proper ways to apply and remove them. Tell him where he can get supplies.

Ensuring proper nutrition can be difficult, but the patient and his family need to know how important proper nutrition is to the healing process. Provide materials on nutrition and maintaining an ideal weight, as appropriate. Show them how to create an easy-to-read chart of care reminders for a wall at home.

EXPERT TIPS

Pressure ulcer do's and don'ts

With proper skin care and frequent position changes, patients and their caregivers can keep the patient's skin healthy—a crucial element in pressure ulcer prevention. Here are some important do's and don'ts to pass along to patients:

DO...
● Change position at least once every 2 hours while re-clining. Follow a schedule. Lie on your right side, then your left side, then your back, then your stomach (if possible). Use pillows and pads for support. Make small turns between the 2-hour changes.
● Check your skin for signs of pressure ulcers twice daily. Use a mirror to check areas you can't inspect directly, such as the shoulders, tailbone, hips, elbows, heels, and the back of the head. Report breaks in the skin or changes in skin temperature to your doctor.

● Follow the prescribed exercise program, including range-of-motion exercises every 8 hours, or as recommended.
● Eat a well-balanced diet, drink lots of fluids, and strive to maintain the recommended weight.

DON'T...
● Use commercial soaps or skin products that dry or irritate your skin—use oil-free lotions.
● Sleep on wrinkled bed sheets or tuck your covers tightly into the foot of your bed.

Pressure ulcers should be reassessed weekly. Measure progress by the reduction in necrotic tissue and drainage, and the increase in granulation tissue and epithelial growth. Clean, vascularized pressure ulcers should show evidence of healing within 2 weeks. If they don't and the patient has followed the guidelines for nutrition, reposi-tioning, use of support surfaces, and wound care, it's time to reevaluate the care plan.

8

DIABETIC FOOT ULCERS

Diabetes mellitus is a metabolic disorder characterized by hyperglycemia resulting from lack of insulin, lack of insulin effect, or both. Insulin transports glucose into cells, where it's used as fuel or stored as glycogen. Insulin also stimulates protein synthesis and storage of free fatty acids in fat deposits; an insulin deficiency compromises these important functions. Diabetes can begin suddenly or develop insidiously.

High glucose levels caused by diabetes can damage blood vessels and nerves; therefore, patients with diabetes are susceptible to developing foot ulcers caused by nerve damage and poor circulation to the legs and feet. Good diabetes control may help prevent these potentially chronic problems or make them less serious.

Causes

Diabetic neuropathy, pressure and other mechanical forces, and poor circulation can cause foot ulcers in patients with diabetes.

DIABETIC NEUROPATHY
Peripheral neuropathy is the primary cause of diabetic foot ulcer development. Neuropathy is a nerve disorder

that results in impaired or lost function in the tissues served by the affected nerve fibers. In diabetes, neuropathy may be caused by ischemia due to thickening in the tiny blood vessels that supply the nerve or by nerve demyelinization (destruction of the protective myelin sheath surrounding a nerve), which slows the conduction of impulses.

Polyneuropathy, or damage to multiple types of nerves, is the most common form of neuropathy in patients with diabetes. In the foot, a trineuropathy develops that includes:

■ loss of sensation
■ loss of motor function
■ loss of autonomic functions (the autonomic nervous system controls smooth muscles, glands, and visceral organs). (See *Understanding diabetic trineuropathy,* pages 210 and 211.)

Typically, impairment affects the feet and hands first and then progresses toward the knees and elbows, respectively. This presentation is called a *stocking-and-glove distribution.*

As sensory nerves degenerate and die (sensory neuropathy), the patient experiences a burning or "pins-and-needles" sensation that might worsen at night.

As sensation declines, the patient risks foot injury. Impaired sensation prevents the patient from feeling stimuli, such as pain and pressure that normally warn of impending tissue damage. Anything from stepping on something sharp to wearing ill-fitting shoes can result in foot injury because the patient can't feel the damage occurring.

As motor nerves degenerate and die (motor neuropathy), muscles in the limbs atrophy, especially the intrinsic muscles of the feet, which causes footdrop and structural deformities. These degenerative changes increase the pa-

Understanding diabetic trineuropathy

Uncontrolled diabetes commonly results in a trineuropathy (three concurrent neuropathies) that dramatically increases the patient's risk of developing diabetic foot ulcers.

SENSORY NEUROPATHY
In sensory neuropathy, ischemia or demyelinization (see illustration below) causes nerve death or deterioration. When this occurs, the patient no longer feels painful stimuli and, therefore, can no longer respond appropriately.

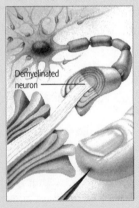

Demyelinated neuron

MOTOR NEUROPATHY
In motor neuropathy, muscles deep in the sole of the foot atrophy, resulting in increased arch height and clawed toes. In addition, the fat pad that normally covers the metatarsal heads migrates toward the

toes, exposing the metatarsal heads to more pressure and increasing pressure ulcer risk. The risk is high for the upper surfaces of clawed toes as well, especially if the patient has poorly fitted shoes.

The illustration below shows the degenerative changes in the foot resulting from motor neuropathy. Shading indicates the areas where ulcers are most likely to develop.

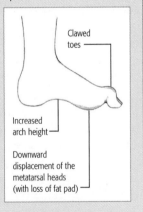

Clawed toes

Increased arch height

Downward displacement of the metatarsal heads (with loss of fat pad)

AUTONOMIC NEUROPATHY
In uncontrolled diabetes, autonomic neuropathy inhibits or

Understanding diabetic trineuropathy
(*continued*)

destroys the sympathetic component of the autonomic nervous system, which controls vasoconstriction in peripheral blood vessels. The resulting free flow of blood to the lower limbs and feet may cause osteopenia (reduction of bone volume) in foot and ankle bones.

In Charcot disease (neuropathic osteoarthropathy), the bones weakened by osteopenia suffer fractures that the patient doesn't feel due to sensory neuropathy. Over time, this process causes bony dissolution that culminates with the collapse of the midfoot into a rocker bottom deformity (see illustration). Patients with Charcot disease are placed on non–weight-bearing status until inflammation subsides.

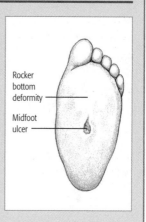

Midfoot ulcers resulting from increased plantar pressures over the rocker bottom deformity heal slower than ulcers on the forefoot.

tient's risk of stumbling or falling and further damaging the foot.

As autonomic nerves degenerate and die (autonomic neuropathy), sweat and sebaceous glands malfunction and skin on the patient's feet dries and cracks. If fissures develop, the risk of infection increases.

MECHANICAL FORCES

Mechanical forces involved in diabetic ulcer generation include pressure, friction, and shear.

Pressure

Sensory neuropathy places a patient at increased risk for diabetic foot ulcers caused by pressure—especially a patient who's confined to a bed or wheelchair. Such a patient can suffer damage simply by letting his feet rest for too long on a bed or a wheelchair footrest. Impaired sensation prevents the patient from feeling the discomfort that results from remaining in one position too long.

As with pressure ulcers, areas over bony prominences are the most common places for diabetic foot ulcers, including:

■ metatarsal heads
■ great toe
■ heel.

Friction and shear

Although pressure is the major mechanical force at work in the development of diabetic ulcers, it isn't the only one. Friction and shear can also cause damage. A loose shoe rubbing against the foot or a foot sliding across a bed sheet can cause friction damage.

Shearing forces build up when damp skin sticks to a surface while the underlying bone and tissue move. For example, the skin of a sweating foot can cling to a shoe while the underlying tissues slide beneath the skin.

PERIPHERAL VASCULAR DISEASE

Peripheral vascular disease (PVD), a common problem in patients with diabetes, impairs the healing process of existing ulcers and may contribute to neuropathy. In PVD, atherosclerosis narrows the peripheral arteries, slowly re-

How atherosclerosis impairs circulation

In atherosclerosis, fatty deposits (cholesterol) and fibrous plaques accumulate along the walls of the arteries, narrowing the lumen and reducing the artery's elasticity. Thrombi (blood clots) form on the roughened surface of plaques and may grow large enough to block the artery's lumen.

In diabetes, the arterial damage caused by atherosclerosis reduces blood flow to the lower limbs and to the nerves that innervate them. In addition to promoting ulcer development, poor perfusion slows the healing process for existing ulcers and impedes circulation of systemic antibiotics to infected areas.

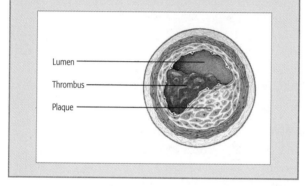

ducing the flow of blood to the limbs. (See *How atherosclerosis impairs circulation.*) As perfusion decreases, the risks of ischemia and tissue necrosis increase.

Patient care

Optimal care of diabetic foot ulcers includes a knowledge of the patient's history, regular foot examinations, and special testing.

HISTORY

Knowledge of the patient's history is vital to caring for diabetic foot ulcers. In addition to the basic information elicited during a traditional patient history, find out about:

- date of onset of diabetes
- management measures
- medications
- other diagnosed problems
- status and history of diagnosed neuropathy
- allergies, especially skin reactions
- tobacco and alcohol use
- recent changes in activity level
- glycemic control
- lipid panel
- date and location of previous ulcerations
- date the current ulcer was first noticed
- the way in which the ulcer occurred
- type and quality of pain.

PHYSICAL EXAMINATION

Use a holistic approach when performing the physical examination. Remember that the patient's overall physical health and state of mind affect wound healing.

The general physical examination evaluates the patient's musculoskeletal, neurologic, vascular, and integumentary systems to provide perspective for evaluating the condition of the lower limbs.

Note these aspects of the patient's musculoskeletal system:

- posture
- gait
- strength, flexibility, and endurance
- range of motion.

Note these aspects of the patient's neurologic system:

- balance

- reflexes
- sensory function.

Note these aspects of the patient's vascular system:

- posterior tibial and dorsalis pedis pulses
- ankle-brachial index (ABI); this may not always be reliable in a patient with diabetes due to calcification in the microvasculature.

Note these aspects of the patient's integumentary system:

- texture
- temperature
- color
- appendages (hair, sweat glands, sebaceous glands, nails).

Foot examination

An evaluation of the patient's feet is central to detecting and caring for diabetic foot ulcers. Check these high-risk areas of the feet for existing or impending ulcers:

- plantar surfaces (soles) of the toes
- tips of the toes
- between the toes
- side of the foot's sole.

Wound characteristics depend on where the wound occurs on the foot. (See *Features of diabetic foot ulcers*, page 216.) Characteristics of surrounding skin may include:

- calluses (considered prewounds)
- blood blisters (hemorrhage beneath a callus)
- erythema, indicating inflammation or infection
- induration (hardened edges)
- skin fissures (portals for bacterial entry)
- dry, scaly skin.

Features of diabetic foot ulcers

In diabetic foot ulcers, characteristic features depend on the location of the ulcer.

ULCER LOCATION	CLINICAL FEATURES
Plantar surface	Even wound margins
Great toe	Deep wound bed
Metatarsal head	Dry or low to moderate exudate
Heel	Low to moderate exudate
Tip or top of toe	Pale granulation with ischemia or bright-red, friable granulation tissue with infection

SPECIAL TESTING

Special tests provide a clearer picture of the health of the lower leg and foot. These tests evaluate pressure, neurologic function, and perfusion. The results provide insight into the mechanism of injury, condition of the wound bed and surrounding tissue, prognosis for healing, and required treatment interventions. Although as an LPN you won't be required to perform these tests, a basic understanding of them may help with patient teaching.

Musculoskeletal tests

Harris mat prints and computerized pressure mapping are special musculoskeletal tests that provide information about the plantar pressures of the foot.

HARRIS MAT PRINTS

Pressure over bony prominences is one cause of diabetic foot ulcers. A simple method for determining where areas of increased pressure are on the sole of the foot is to use an ink mat.

Ink is placed on the sole of the patient's foot. He then steps on the uninked top surface of a mat, placing equal weight on each foot. The impression on the mat or sheet of paper shows relative areas of pressure under the patient's foot. Darker areas on the grid indicate high-pressure areas. When a dynamic impression is required, the patient slowly walks across the mat to create the impression.

High-pressure areas usually correlate with calluses (prewounds) or existing wounds. The test results help guide the choice of special off-loading devices, which help relieve pressure when the patient stands or walks.

COMPUTERIZED PRESSURE MAPPING
Computerized pressure mapping devices test pressures while the patient is wearing a shoe and when he's barefoot. The approach is similar to that used to create Harris mat prints, but in this test a computer maps the pressures and displays the results on a printout. A color gradient illustrates relative pressure, with red and orange indicating areas of highest pressure.

Neurologic tests
Neurologic tests for the legs and feet include:
- testing deep tendon reflexes (DTRs)
- vibration perception testing with a tuning fork or biothesiometer
- Semmes-Weinstein monofilament testing for protective sensation.

TESTING DTRS

Peripheral neuropathy causes a decrease in DTRs. Decreased DTRs correlate with muscular atrophy, usually the intrinsic muscles of the foot in a patient with diabetes.

TUNING FORK TEST

In this test, a tuning fork is used to assess peripheral nerve function and help identify and quantify neuropathy. The results of both limbs are compared to assess neurologic function.

BIOTHESIOMETER

A biothesiometer is used to assess vibratory perception threshold. It provides a better quantitative measurement of vibratory sense than the tuning fork. Individuals with sensory neuropathy have impaired vibratory perception thresholds.

SEMMES-WEINSTEIN TEST

The Semmes-Weinstein test helps determine the level of protective sensation in the feet. While the patient's eyes are closed he is asked to identify when and where the skin has been touched with a Semmes-Weinstein monofilament. As protective sensation decreases, pressure tends to increase, as does the patient's risk of ulcers at these points.

Vascular tests

Vascular tests help assess circulation in the lower extremities. These tests include pulse palpation, ABI, and toe pressures.

PULSE PALPATION

Initial assessment of limb perfusion includes palpation of the dorsalis pedis, posterior tibial, popliteal, and femoral

Assessing pulse strength

When assessing the amplitude of a pulse, rate the strength on a numerical scale or use a specific descriptive term. You can use this scale to rate the patient's pulse.

RATING	PULSE CHARACTERISTIC
0	No palpable pulse
+1	Weak or thready pulse: hard to feel, easily obliterated by slight finger pressure
+2	Normal pulse: easily palpable, obliterated by strong finger pressure
+3	Bounding pulse: readily palpable, forceful, not easily obliterated by finger pressure

pulses. If it's hard to palpate a pulse due to edema, a Doppler ultrasound is used, which produces an audible signal that coincides with the pulse.

The transducer is held at a 45-degree angle to the skin and the audio of the beats is evaluated. The results provide a general idea of the circulation to each level of the leg. A palpable dorsalis pedis pulse is roughly equivalent to 80 mm Hg, which is adequate for healing most diabetic wounds. (See *Assessing pulse strength*.)

ANKLE-BRACHIAL INDEX
PVD and resulting poor perfusion are common problems for patients with diabetes. Poor perfusion increases the patient's likelihood of developing ulcers and reduces the speed with which existing ulcers heal. ABI is used with other vascular tests to determine and monitor the patient's risk of ischemia in the area of the ankle. ABI is a ratio of

systolic blood pressure in the brachial artery in the arm to systolic blood pressure measured in the dorsalis pedis artery in the ankle.

TOE PRESSURES

Toe pressures may be a more sensitive indicator of changes in vascular integrity in the distal areas of the foot. Toe pressures are measured in the same manner as arm blood pressures, except that a much smaller, specialized cuff is used for the toe. Due to the tiny arteries in digits, the corresponding arterial pressures are lower than those measured in an arm or leg. Typical pressure in the toe is about 70% of systolic values obtained in the arm.

Classification

Diabetic foot ulcers are classified according to depth, presence of ischemia, and presence of infection, depending on the classification system. The Wagner ulcer grade classification system and the University of Texas wound classification system for diabetic foot ulcers are two commonly used classification systems.

WAGNER ULCER GRADE CLASSIFICATION SYSTEM

The original Wagner ulcer grade classification system considers depth of penetration; however, it doesn't allow for the assessment of infection at all tissue levels. A modified version of the Wagner classification system adds levels that take into account infection and ischemia. (See *Using the Wagner ulcer grade classification system*.)

Using the Wagner ulcer grade classification system

In the Wagner ulcer grade classification system, less complex ulcers receive lower scores; more complex ulcers receive higher scores. Ulcers with higher scores may require surgical intervention or amputation.

GRADE	CHARACTERISTICS
0	• Preulcer lesion • Healed ulcer • Presence of bony deformity
1	• Superficial ulcer without subcutaneous tissue involvement
2	• Penetration through the subcutaneous tissue; may expose bone, tendon, ligament, or joint capsule
3	• Osteitis, abscess, or osteomyelitis
4	• Gangrene of a digit
5	• Gangrene requiring foot amputation

Adapted with permission from Wagner, F.W., Jr. "The Diabetic Foot," *Orthopedics* 10:163-72, 1987. © Slack Incorporated.

UNIVERSITY OF TEXAS WOUND CLASSIFICATION SYSTEM

The University of Texas wound classification system for diabetic foot ulcers takes tissue infection and ischemia into consideration and provides a more detailed breakdown of classifications than the Wagner system. (See *Using the University of Texas wound classification system*, page 222.)

Using the University of Texas wound classification system

The University of Texas wound classification system provides a detailed categorization of diabetic foot ulcers. This system allows for the consideration of infection and ischemia.

STAGE	GRADE 0	GRADE I	GRADE II	GRADE III
A	Preulcerative or postulcerative foot at risk for further ulceration	Superficial ulcer without tendon, capsule, or bone involvement	Ulcer penetrating to tendon or joint capsule	Ulcer penetrating to bone
B	Presence of infection	Presence of infection	Presence of infection	Presence of infection
C	Presence of ischemia	Presence of ischemia	Presence of ischemia	Presence of ischemia
D	Presence of infection and ischemia	Presence of infection and ischemia	Presence of infection and ischemia	Presence of infection and ischemia

Adapted with permission from Armstrong, D.G., et al. "Treatment-based Classification System for Assessment and Care of Diabetic Feet," *JAPMA* 86(7): 311-16, 1996.

Complications

The most common complications that impede the healing of diabetic foot ulcers include:
- multiple comorbidities, including PVD—cause a number of problems that increase the risk of ulceration and reduce the likelihood of speedy healing
- uncontrolled hyperglycemia—commonly signals infection and inhibits the immune system, particularly the scavenging function of neutrophils

■ psychosocial problems, such as depression and poverty—profoundly affect the patient's nutritional status, which in turn affects the body's ability to prevent ulcers and heal existing wounds.

Any of these complications can cause a wound to become chronic.

INFECTION

Infection is a common complication in diabetic foot ulcers. An infection in the wound or elsewhere consumes protein needed for healing and interferes directly by damaging the wound bed.

Uncontrollable glucose level or hyperglycemia may be the first sign of infection because patients with diabetes commonly fail to demonstrate the typical systemic responses. An infection in the wound bed commonly causes friable (easy to bleed), bright-red granulation tissue.

Osteomyelitis or bone infection is common in deep wounds. A quick and reliable method for determining whether osteomyelitis is present in a diabetic ulcer bed is to palpate for bone. A palpable bone usually indicates osteomyelitis. However, osteomyelitis may be difficult to distinguish from acute Charcot neuropathic osteoarthropathy. The best way to differentiate between the two is to culture a bone fragment from the wound bed.

Infections fall into two categories: limb-threatening or non–limb-threatening. Non–limb-threatening infections tend to be superficial infections involving tissues within 2 cm of the wound margin. In this type of infection, no significant tissue ischemia is present and bone isn't palpable in the wound bed. Non–limb-threatening infection can be treated with topical antimicrobials, sharp debridement, and wound cleaning once or twice per day.

In contrast, limb-threatening infection involves tissue more than 2 cm from the wound margin, palpable bone in the wound bed, and tissue ischemia. Hospitalization and surgical debridement of infected bone and soft tissues is requisite. Unless the infected bone is fully resected (surgically removed), the patient requires 4 to 8 weeks of I.V. antibiotic therapy.

Diabetic foot ulcer care

Successful healing depends on proper wound cleaning and dressing and off-loading (relieving pressure). Topical antimicrobials, debridement, biotherapies, and surgery may also be included in the care plan.

WOUND CLEANING

Wound cleaning is a fundamental step in the healing process. Necrotic tissue is a reservoir for bacteria and inhibits wound healing.

Flushing the wound bed with normal saline solution is the best method of cleaning a diabetic foot ulcer. Most commercial wound cleaners are somewhat toxic to cells in the wound bed, and their use can slow healing. Use clean, warm water and mild soap to clean the surrounding skin.

Cleaning the wound bed can be made easier by using bulb syringes, syringes with angiocatheters, aerosolized saline in a canister, pulsatile lavage with suction, and whirlpool. (For more information on wound cleaning, see chapter 4, Basic wound care procedures.)

WOUND DRESSINGS

Moist wound therapy speeds healing in diabetic foot ulcers. Dressings that maintain the necessary wound environment include:

- alginates
- transparent films
- foams

- hydrocolloids
- hydrogels
- collagen-based dressings
- composites (combinations of the other dressings)
- hydrofiber dressings
- silver-impregnated dressings.

Choice of dressing depends on the condition of the ulcer. Diabetic foot ulcers tend to produce low to moderate drainage. If the wound bed is dry, however, it needs a dressing that adds moisture. Either amorphous hydrogels or sheet hydrogels can help in this case. Hydrogel sheets are more cost-effective but don't work as well in deeper wounds. For deep or tunneling ulcers that require packing, hydrogel-impregnated gauze is an excellent alternative to amorphous hydrogels and costs less. All hydrogel dressings add moisture to the wound bed—they're as much as 95% water themselves. Hydrogels also encourage autolytic debridement. (See *Types of dressings for diabetic foot ulcers*, page 226.)

OFF-LOADING

Off-loading from plantar tissues is the cornerstone of diabetic neuropathy treatment as well as prevention for those patients at risk for recurrent breakdown. Off-loading seeks to control, limit, or remove all intrinsic and extrinsic factors that increase plantar pressures. Examples of intrinsic risk factors include faulty biomechanics in the foot or the presence of a bony deformity. Extrinsic risk factors include trauma, ill-fitting shoes, or maintaining a position for too long, allowing the damaging effects of pressure to build up—for example, lying supine in bed or resting a heel against the footrest of a wheelchair.

Off-loading is particularly important because patients with diabetic neuropathy can't feel the growing discom-

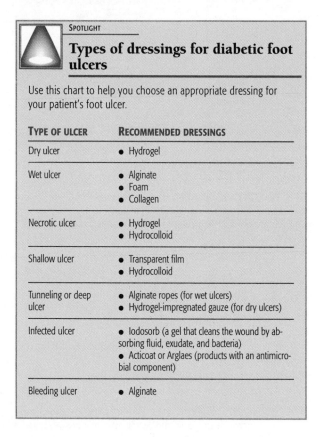

SPOTLIGHT
Types of dressings for diabetic foot ulcers

Use this chart to help you choose an appropriate dressing for your patient's foot ulcer.

TYPE OF ULCER	RECOMMENDED DRESSINGS
Dry ulcer	• Hydrogel
Wet ulcer	• Alginate • Foam • Collagen
Necrotic ulcer	• Hydrogel • Hydrocolloid
Shallow ulcer	• Transparent film • Hydrocolloid
Tunneling or deep ulcer	• Alginate ropes (for wet ulcers) • Hydrogel-impregnated gauze (for dry ulcers)
Infected ulcer	• Iodosorb (a gel that cleans the wound by absorbing fluid, exudate, and bacteria) • Acticoat or Arglaes (products with an antimicrobial component)
Bleeding ulcer	• Alginate

fort that precedes tissue damage. Off-loading pressure prevents or limits the kind of tissue damage that causes ulcers to form.

Nonsurgical off-loading techniques

Off-loading can be accomplished using nonsurgical or surgical interventions. Nonsurgical interventions include therapeutic footwear, possibly with rocker soles; custom orthotics; and walking casts. When considering a device for a patient, keep in mind that using a device can increase the patient's risk of falling. If this is true for your patient, provide instruction on fall prevention.

SHOES

Good shoes are important. For a patient with no loss of protective sensation, this may equate to a comfortable, well-fitting pair of tennis shoes. A patient with recurring ulcers and severe foot deformities needs a custom-molded shoe. Common design features of therapeutic footwear include:

- soft, breathable leather that conforms to foot deformities
- high tops for ankle stability
- rocker soles and bottoms for pressure and pain relief across the plantar metatarsal heads
- a toe box with extra depth and width to accommodate deformities, such as claw toes and hallux valgus (displacement of the great toe toward the other toes)
- flared lateral soles for stability.

(See *Types of therapeutic shoe modifications,* page 228.)

CUSTOM ORTHOTIC DEVICES

Custom orthotic devices are shoe inserts that serve various functions based on the patient's needs. In general, custom orthotic devices relieve pressure, reduce shearing force and friction, and cushion the foot against shocks. If necessary, custom orthotic devices also accommodate the patient's foot deformities.

WALKING CASTS

Walking casts range from total contact casts to splints and walkers.

A total contact cast is the top-of-the-line in care for uninfected diabetic ulcers on the plantar surface of the foot. Total contact casts are custom made for each patient

Types of therapeutic shoe modifications

These illustrations show the modifications in custom shoes that can improve stability and accommodate the deformities that affect many patients with diabetes.

HIGH TOP

LATERAL FLARE

ROCKER SOLE

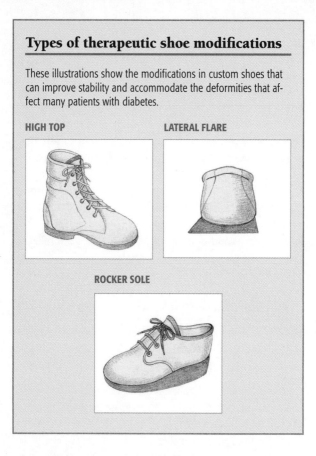

by a health care professional, typically a physical therapist or orthotist. Inside the cast, padding is fitted over bony areas of the ankle and leg that are at risk for pressure ulcers. A plaster shell reinforced with plaster splints covers the padding. Fiberglass covers the plaster to lend rigidity and additional strength. The cast includes a sturdy walking heel for ambulation. The cast is molded to fit snugly to prevent the foot from sliding inside the cast, reducing shearing force over the plantar surface.

A patient with an infected diabetic ulcer isn't a candidate for a total contact cast because a cast makes daily assessment, cleaning, and antimicrobial therapy impossible. In addition, inflammation and edema can cause a buildup of pressure within the cast and subsequent tissue damage. In the case of infection, a removable off-loading device is recommended.

Splints and walkers have cushioned inserts with an outer shell of fiberglass or copolymer. Several splint and walker options are available. Splints and walkers have some advantages of their own. For example, they allow easy inspection of the ulcer. In addition, off-loading modifications can be accomplished relatively easy by changing the type of walker or splint in use. However, these devices also have disadvantages. First and foremost, they don't provide the same degree of pressure and shear relief as a total contact cast. Also, for these therapies to work, the patient must be committed to using the device—a patient can always take off a splint or choose not to use a walker on any given day.

Surgical interventions

Surgical off-loading procedures include surgical dissection of the wound bed and pressure-inducing bony tissue deformities. Pressure over bony prominences compresses and occludes blood vessels, causing ischemia. Resecting bone deformities reduces peak plantar pressures. This type of surgery is called *curative surgery* because it removes the pathologic tissue. Examples of curative surgery include exostectomy, digital arthroplasty, bone and joint resections, and partial calcanectomy.

TOPICAL ANTIMICROBIALS

Routine wound cleaning abates much of the surface microbial population. However, applying a topical antimicrobial directly to the wound bed can help control microorganisms in the wound bed and improve healing. Commonly used topical antimicrobials include:

- bacitracin
- metronidazole (MetroGel)
- mupirocin (Bactroban)
- silver sulfadiazine (Silvadene).

Some microorganisms are resistant to certain topical agents. Furthermore, recent findings indicate that neomycin-containing products, such as Neosporin, can cause allergic reactions. Consequently, these are no longer recommended for ulcer treatment.

More recent wound care antimicrobials include Iodosorb gel, Iodoflex pad, Arglaes antimicrobial barrier, and Acticoat. These products contain iodine or silver, which kills or inhibits microbes. The active ingredients are released slowly in concentrations that are toxic to microbes but not to important cells, such as fibroblasts, in the wound bed. As an added benefit, research seems to indicate that microbes aren't as likely to develop resistance to this new generation of products.

DEBRIDEMENT

Debriding necrotic and nonviable tissue, foreign matter, and microbes from the wound bed expedites wound healing. Surgical debridement, the most effective method of debridement, is required in cases of osteomyelitis or when the wound involves a deep abscess or spreading tissue infection. Sharp debridement, which can be performed at the bedside, is an option when surgery isn't necessary or the patient is a poor surgical candidate. Topical proteolytic enzymes can be applied to wound tissue to augment debridement between sessions. (For more information on wound debridement, see chapter 4, Basic wound care procedures.)

BIOTHERAPIES

Growth factors and living skin equivalents are two forms of biotherapy that may be included in the care plan for a patient with a diabetic foot ulcer.

Growth factors

Growth factors orchestrate healing in the wound bed. One factor in particular—platelet-derived growth factor (PDGF)—is called the *master factor*. PDGF plays a central role by stimulating chemotaxis and the proliferation of neutrophils, fibroblasts, and monocytes. Becaplermin (Regranex Gel 0.01%) is the only PDGF-based product approved by the Food and Drug Administration for diabetic foot ulcers. In clinical trials, it has shown an increase in wound closure rates. However, this therapy also relies on an adequate vascular supply and proper wound bed preparation. Its use on superficial diabetic foot ulcers isn't recommended.

Living skin equivalents

Living skin equivalents are products composed of living cells and a matrix, or scaffolding, which serves as the extracellular medium. These products act as interactive wound coverings, providing growth factors and other needed molecules. Dermagraft is one example of a living skin equivalent. It has viable fibroblasts that enhance wound healing rates in diabetic ulcers. Graftskin (Apligraf), another living skin equivalent, also accelerates wound healing.

Prevention

Diabetic ulcer prevention starts with identifying the patient's risk factors and then teaching him how to eliminate or minimize these risks.

IDENTIFYING RISKS

Identifying your patient's risk factors is an important part of prevention. Loss of sensation is the single biggest risk factor, but it isn't the only one. Here's a list of risk factors for diabetic ulcers compiled by the American College of Foot and Ankle Surgeons:

- structural foot deformity (such as claw toes, rocker bottom, or hallux vagus)
- trauma and improperly fitted shoes
- calluses
- prior history of ulcerations or amputation
- prolonged, elevated pressure on areas of tissue
- limited joint mobility
- uncontrolled hyperglycemia
- prolonged history of diabetes
- blindness or partial sight
- chronic renal disease
- advanced age.

PATIENT TEACHING

The next step in prevention is patient education, including teaching about ulcer care and prevention and the importance of controlling diabetes, including the consequences of not controlling it—for example, teaching that poorly controlled blood glucose levels can lead to peripheral neuropathy and vascular damage. Research indicates that tight glycemic control reduces the frequency and severity of neuropathy in individuals with type 1 diabetes. Similar findings have been shown for individuals with type 2 diabetes.

Teach the patient proper foot care and steps to prevent ulcers, including daily examinations, skin washing and maintenance techniques, toenail care, and exercise. Also instruct the patient on how to choose proper socks and shoes. (See *Teaching proper foot care*.)

Teaching proper foot care

With proper skin care and frequent position changes, patients and their caregivers can keep the patient's skin healthy—a crucial element in pressure ulcer prevention. Here are some important do's and don'ts to pass along to patients.

FOOT CARE
- Check feet daily for injury or pressure areas (a long-handled mirror can help).
- Wash feet with a mild soap and dry thoroughly between toes.
- Check bath water to make sure it isn't too hot (test water with your elbow, if able; otherwise, use a thermometer or ask a family member to help).
- Apply a moisturizing cream (petroleum jelly is inexpensive and effective) to prevent dry, cracking skin on the feet and to balance skin pH. Don't apply moisturizer between the toes.
- Cut toenails off squarely; see a podiatrist if they're dystrophic (deformed and thickened).
- Avoid being barefoot—the risk of injury is too great.

SOCKS
- Use silver ion-lined socks for fungus control.
- Wear white or light-colored socks so that bleeding from

trauma can be detected quickly.
- Wear natural fiber socks— they breathe better than synthetics.
- Wear socks that wick perspiration away from feet to prevent maceration.
- Use diabetic padded socks for shear and friction control.

SHOES
- Wear well-fitting shoes; avoid shoes that are too tight or loose.
- Wear shoes that breathe to reduce maceration and fungal infections.
- Wear new shoes for short periods (under 1 hour) each day initially; gradually increase the time as your feet adjust.
- Wear professionally fitted shoes if deformities are present or you have a history of ulceration.
- Wash shoes, if possible, to destroy microorganisms.
- Check shoes before putting them on to make sure nothing fell in that could cause harm.

White cotton-blend socks are the best choice for a patient with diabetes. Cotton-blended socks wick away moisture and allow air to circulate around the foot. White socks vividly show blood or exudate from an injury or ulcer that the patient may not feel. Regardless of the material, socks should always be nonconstricting and seamless over bony prominences. Socks with added padding can provide additional cushioning as well as some protection from shearing force.

Successful prevention programs for diabetic ulcers begin with health promotion. Your patient is at the center of the health care team—all activity focuses on his health needs. In this team, the patient plays an active role in setting personal health care goals, working in partnership with the health care team, who can help him achieve those goals.

Most patients with diabetes have multiple disorders, requiring a series of interventions involving many health disciplines—nurses, physicians, physical therapists, occupational therapists, nutritionists, podiatrists, endocrinologists, psychologists, diabetes educators, prosthetists or orthotists, and social workers.

9

WOUND CARE PRODUCTS

Over time, wound care has developed from a fairly rudimentary practice that focused primarily on care of the injury to a process that considers the complexities of the patient's general health, possible underlying disease, and specific wound characteristics. As wound care knowledge increased, so did the number and types of products available to aid healing.

In this chapter, we'll look at basic and advanced wound care products and the indications, advantages, and disadvantages of each. Keep in mind that the products discussed here are tools that can help promote full healing, but they aren't the only tools you need. Unless problems such as malnutrition, circulatory disorders, and patient knowledge deficits are addressed, the healing process halts. In addition, no wound care dressing or topical agent can compensate for an incomplete wound evaluation. In short, let the findings of a thorough evaluation guide your wound care product selection. (See *Selecting wound care products,* page 236.)

Given the number of products available now, it's hard to believe that there could be anything new around the corner. But new products arrive almost daily, and others are updated or improved regularly. Because the quality of the care that you provide depends on your level of knowl-

Selecting wound care products

When selecting wound care products, ask these important questions:

● Which companies have contracts to supply wound care products to your facility? (Learn about these products first.)

● What's the simplest method of closing the wound? Which is most cost effective?

● Can the patient afford the supplies he needs? (Simple and affordable aren't necessarily synonymous.) If not, is financial assistance available?

● Who provides wound care at home? If the patient can't perform this important task, can family members or friends? Is home health care an option? If so, is the patient eligible?

● What caused the wound, and how can the cause best be alleviated? (This is especially important when treating chronic wounds; less so when treating acute wounds.)

● How often does the dressing need to be changed? (It takes several hours—at least 8 hours—for a wound to achieve homeostasis after a dressing change. Therefore, less often is better.)

● How much drainage is present?

● Does the wound need more moisture?

● Should the wound be debrided? If so, which method is best for the patient?

● After cleaning and drying, does the wound (not the dressing) have an unpleasant odor? Do you suspect infection? If so, is a culture warranted?

● Is there tunneling, undermining, or a cavity that needs to be filled?

● Are the wound edges open or closed? (Wound edges must be open for complete healing to occur.)

● How large is the wound? Would it be more cost-effective to use an advanced wound care product to facilitate granulation tissue or closure?

edge, it's imperative that you stay up-to-date by periodically reviewing the products available.

Wound dressings

The most durable wound dressing, gauze has been used for more years than any other material. However, as medical research has afforded a better understanding of wounds and the healing process, medical manufacturers have developed new materials and sophisticated dressing options that better promote healing.

Moisture level, tissue adherence, infection control, and wound dimensions are just some of the factors that affect wound dressing selection. The level of moisture in the wound bed is critical to the success or failure of healing. Consequently, one fundamental way to classify dressings is by their effect on wound moisture: do they add, absorb, or not affect wound moisture? (See *Dressings for specific wound types,* page 238, and *Quick guide to topical therapy,* page 239.)

Although gauze remains a good choice for secondary dressings, it no longer represents the most effective choice for a primary dressing. A number of other dressings are available, including:

- alginate
- biological
- collagen
- composite
- contact layer
- foam
- hydrocolloid
- hydrogel
- specialty absorptive
- transparent film.

ALGINATE DRESSINGS

Made from seaweed, these nonwoven, absorptive dressings are available as soft, white, sterile pads or ropes. Algi-

Dressings for specific wound types

Some dressings absorb moisture from a wound bed, whereas others add moisture to it. Use this chart to quickly determine the category of dressing that's appropriate for your patient.

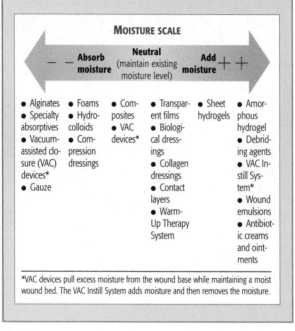

MOISTURE SCALE

Absorb moisture		**Neutral** (maintain existing moisture level)	**Add moisture**	
• Alginates • Specialty absorptives • Vacuum-assisted closure (VAC) devices* • Gauze	• Foams • Hydrocolloids • Compression dressings	• Composites • VAC devices*	• Transparent films • Biological dressings • Collagen dressings • Contact layers • Warm-Up Therapy System	• Sheet hydrogels	• Amorphous hydrogel • Debriding agents • VAC Instill System* • Wound emulsions • Antibiotic creams and ointments

*VAC devices pull excess moisture from the wound base while maintaining a moist wound bed. The VAC Instill System adds moisture and then removes the moisture.

nate dressings absorb excessive exudate and may be used on infected wounds. As the dressing absorbs exudate, it turns into a gel that keeps the wound bed moist and promotes healing. Alginates, which are nonadhesive and nonocclusive, promote autolysis. Use alginate dressings on wounds with moderate to heavy drainage.

Examples of alginate products include:

■ AlgiSite M
■ FyBron Calcium Alginate Dressing

Quick guide to topical therapy

Use this quick guide when choosing a topical therapy to treat a pressure ulcer.

THERAPY	STAGE OF PRESSURE ULCER
Alginates	Draining II, III, IV
Continuous moist gauze	II, III, IV
Enzymes	III, IV (with necrosis)
Foams	II, III, IV
Hydrocolloids	I, II, III
Hydrogels	II, III
Transparent films	I, II, III
Wet to dry gauze	III, IV (with necrosis)

- KALTOSTAT Wound Dressing
- Polymem Calcium Alginate Dressing
- SeaSorb Alginate Dressing
- Sorbsan Topical Wound Dressing
- Tegagen HG Alginate Dressing.

Alginate dressings are beneficial because they:
- hold 7 to 10 times their weight in fluid
- may be cut to fit wound dimensions
- may be layered for more absorption
- come in ropes that are useful for deep wound packing.

However, alginate dressings:
- may require irrigation when being removed
- require secondary dressings

■ can't be used on third-degree burns
■ may dehydrate the wound bed of a dryer wound.

BIOLOGICAL DRESSINGS

Biological dressings are temporary dressings that function similarly to skin grafts. They may be made from amnionic or chorionic membranes, woven from manmade fibers, harvested from animals (usually pigs), or harvested from cadavers. These dressings are good only for temporary use because the body eventually rejects them. If rejection occurs before the underlying wound heals, the dressing must be replaced with a skin graft.

Examples of biological dressings include:
■ Hyalofill BioPolyMeric Wound Dressing
■ Inerpan
■ Oasis.

Biological dressings should be used as temporary dressings for skin grafting donor sites and burns.

Biological dressings are beneficial because they:
■ may shorten healing times
■ prevent infection and fluid loss
■ ease patient discomfort.

However, biological dressings:
■ are relatively expensive
■ may cause allergic reactions
■ may require secondary dressings.

COLLAGEN DRESSINGS

Collagen dressings, which are made with bovine or avian collagen, accelerate wound healing by encouraging the organization of new collagen fibers and granulation tissue. Examples of collagen dressings include:
■ FIBRACOL PLUS Collagen Wound Dressing with Alginate
■ Matrix Collagen Wound Dressing

- SkinTemp Collagen Dressing
- WOUN'DRES Collagen Hydrogel.

   Collagen dressings are beneficial because they:
- can be used on chronic, clean, nonhealing, granulated wound beds
- are available in gel, granule, and sheet forms
- may contain alginate.

   However, collagen dressings:
- may cause an allergic reaction if the patient is sensitive to bovine or avian products
- require secondary dressings
- aren't appropriate for third-degree burns or on wounds with dry beds.

COMPOSITE DRESSINGS

Composite dressings are hybrids that combine two or more types of dressings into one. For example, a three-layer composite dressing can include a bacterial barrier; an absorbent foam, a hydrocolloid, or a hydrogel layer; and an adherent or a nonadherent outer layer. Examples of composite dressings include:

- Aquacel Hydrofiber Dressing
- COVADERM Plus
- Microdon Soft Cloth Adhesive Wound Dressing
- SOFSORB Wound Dressing
- Tegaderm Composite Dressing
- Versiva.

   Composite dressings can be used as the primary or secondary dressings on wounds with light to moderate drainage. They can also be used to protect peripheral and central I.V. lines.

   Composite dressings are beneficial because they:
- are all-in-one dressings that come in various combinations depending on the patient's wound care needs
- are available in multiple sizes and shapes

■ may have an extended dressing life, thereby reducing the number of dressing changes.

However, composite dressings:

■ can't manage heavily draining wounds
■ lose some of the integrity of the dressing when cut
■ can't be used on third-degree burns.

CONTACT LAYER DRESSINGS

Contact layer dressings are single layers of woven or perforated material suitable for direct contact with the wound's surface. The nonadherent contact layer prevents other dressings from sticking to the surface of the wound. Examples of contact layer dressings include:

■ Conformant 2 Wound Veil
■ Mepitel
■ Profore Wound Contact Layer
■ Telfa Clear.

Contact layer dressings are beneficial because they:

■ allow the flow of drainage to a secondary dressing while preventing that dressing from adhering to the wound
■ decrease the pain experienced during dressing changes
■ can be cut-to-fit or overlap the wound edges.

However, contact layer dressings:

■ require a secondary dressing
■ are contraindicated for use on third-degree burns and infected wounds.

FOAM DRESSINGS

Foam dressings are spongelike polymer dressings that provide a moist wound environment. These dressings are somewhat absorptive and may include an adhesive border.

Examples of foam dressing include:

■ Allevyn Cavity Wound Dressing

- Curafoam
- Hydrasorb Foam Wound Dressing
- Mepilex
- Sof-foam
- Tielle Hydropolymer Dressing.

Use a foam dressing as a primary or secondary dressing on wounds with minimal to moderate drainage (including around tubes) when a nonadherent surface is important.

Foam dressings are beneficial because they:
- have an adhesive border
- don't require a secondary dressing
- may be used in combination with other products
- can manage heavier drainage as they wick moisture from the wound and allow evaporation
- don't fray around the edges like gauze.

However, foam dressings:
- may stick to the wound base
- can't manage large amounts of drainage
- may cause maceration unless they're changed regularly.

HYDROCOLLOID DRESSINGS

Hydrocolloid dressings are adhesive, moldable wafers made of a carbohydrate-based material; most have a waterproof backing. They're impermeable to oxygen, water, and water vapor, and most provide some degree of absorption. Hydrocolloid dressings turn to gel as they absorb moisture, help maintain a moist wound bed, and promote autolytic debridement.

Examples of hydrocolloid dressings include:
- BandAid Advanced Healing Bandages (available over-the-counter)
- Cutinova
- DuoDERM CGF
- Hydrocol

■ 3M Tegasorb Hydrocolloid Dressing
■ Restore Cx Wound Care Dressing.

Hydrocolloid dressings should be used for wounds with minimal to moderate drainage, including wounds with necrosis or slough. Hydrocolloid sheet dressings may also be used as secondary dressings.

Hydrocolloid dressings are beneficial because they:

■ don't stick to a moist wound base
■ maintain moisture by becoming gel as they absorb drainage
■ may require changing only two to three times each week
■ can be easily removed from the wound base
■ are available in contoured forms for use on specific sites
■ are available in several varieties (sheets, powder, or gel) in thin and traditional thickness.

However, hydrocolloid dressings:

■ may have an odor when removed
■ can't be used on burns or dry wounds
■ can't be used for wounds with anaerobic infections
■ can cause skin stripping when removed
■ can cause maceration or hypergranulation
■ may need to be held in place to maximize adhesion.

HYDROGEL DRESSINGS

Hydrogel dressings are water- or glycerin-based polymer dressings. They're nonadherent, provide limited absorption (some are 96% water themselves), and come as tubes of gel or in flexible sheets. Hydrogel dressings add moisture and promote autolytic debridement.

Examples of hydrogel dressings include:

■ Aquasorb Hydrogel Wound Dressing
■ Carrasyn Gel Wound Dressing with Acemannan Hydrogel

- CURASOL Gel Wound Dressing
- Hypergel
- Phyto Derma Wound Gel
- SAF-Gel Hydrating Dermal Wound Dressing
- TOE-AID Toe and Nail Dressing.

Hydrogel dressings should be used on dry wounds or wounds with minimal drainage.

Hydrogel dressings are beneficial because they:
- come in either sheet or amorphous gel form
- may provide cooling that soothes and eases pain.

However, hydrogel dressings:
- require a secondary dressing (with the gel form)
- are expensive if sterile
- have varying viscosities among brands and according to the product's base (water or glycerin).

SPECIALTY ABSORPTIVE DRESSINGS

Specialty absorptive dressings have multiple layers of a highly absorbent material, such as cotton or rayon. They may have adhesive borders. Various forms are available, including gels, pads, gauze, or pillows.

Examples of specialty absorptive dressings include:
- AQUACEL
- BreakAway Wound Dressing
- Sofsorb Wound Dressing
- TENDERSORB WET-PRUF Abdominal Pads.

A specialty absorptive dressing should be used on infected or noninfected wounds with heavy drainage.

Specialty absorptive dressings are beneficial because they:
- are highly absorptive
- require less frequent changes (in most cases)
- hold up to 33% more moisture than alginates
- are available in a variety of forms.

However, specialty absorptive dressings:

▪ can't be used on burns
▪ can't be used on wounds with little or no drainage.

TRANSPARENT FILM DRESSINGS

Transparent film dressings are clear, adherent, nonabsorptive, polyurethane dressings. They're semipermeable to oxygen and water vapor, but not to water itself. Transparency allows visual inspection of the wound while the dressing is in place. Transparent film dressings maintain a moist wound environment and promote autolysis.

Examples of transparent film dressings include:

▪ BIOCLUSIVE Transparent Dressing
▪ 3M NexCare Waterproof Bandages (available over-the-counter)
▪ 3M Tegaderm Transparent Dressing
▪ OpSite Flexigrid
▪ POLYSKIN II Transparent Dressing.

Transparent film dressings should be used on partial-thickness or shallow full-thickness wounds with minimal exudate and on wounds with eschar (dry, leathery, black necrotic tissue) to promote autolysis.

Transparent film dressings are beneficial because they:

▪ may require less frequent changes
▪ allow you to see the wound without removing the dressing
▪ are adherent but won't stick to the wound
▪ aren't bulky.

However, transparent film dressings:

▪ don't absorb drainage
▪ can strip skin when it's removed.

Wound fillers

Wound fillers, as the name suggests, are specialized dressings used to fill deeper wounds. They're made of various materials and come in many forms, such as pastes, granules, powders, beads, and gels. Wound fillers can add moisture to the wound bed or absorb drainage, depending on the product. Examples of wound fillers include:

■ AcryDerm STRANDS Absorbent Wound Filler
■ Bard Absorption Dressing
■ Catrix Wound Dressing
■ MULTIDEX Maltodextrin Wound Dressing Gel or Powder
■ PolyWic Wound Filler.

Wound fillers are beneficial because they:

■ can be used as a primary dressing on an infected or a noninfected wound with minimal to moderate drainage that requires packing
■ come in various forms and absorptive abilities.

However, wound fillers:

■ can't be used on third-degree burns, on dry wounds, or on wounds with tunnels and sinuses
■ can alarm a sensitive patient because of its wormlike appearance.

Adjunct wound care products

A comprehensive listing of topical skin and wound care aids to complement the function of dressings would require several companion volumes; therefore, only selected products and devices that directly impact a wound's ability to heal will be addressed.

PROVANT WOUND CLOSURE SYSTEM

The Provant Wound Closure System is a noninvasive treatment that uses a radio frequency signal to stimulate healing. A treatment signal is directed 2¾" to 3½" (7 to 9 cm) into the tissues around the wound to induce the proliferation of fibroblasts and epithelial cells as well as the secretion of multiple growth factors. The result is faster healing. Treatment doesn't require removal of existing dressings. Clinical studies indicate that the Provant system is effective in promoting healing, even in cases of chronic, severe pressure ulcers.

The Provant system is beneficial to wounds in the inflammatory phase of healing; it:
■ requires no special training (patients may be able to perform therapy at home)
■ requires only two 30-minute treatments per day (duration is preset in the device so it turns off automatically at the end of a session)
■ can facilitate healing of tunneling and undermining and through necrotic tissue and eschar
■ may be used over existing dressings.

However, the Provant system:
■ can't be used in pregnant women or in patients with cardiac pacemakers
■ won't help heal bone or deep internal organs.

VACUUM-ASSISTED CLOSURE DEVICE

The vacuum-assisted closure (VAC) device uses negative air pressure to promote wound healing. This system consists of a special open-cell polyurethane ether foam dressing cut to the size of the wound, a vacuum tube, and a vacuum pump. One end of the vacuum tube is placed over the foam dressing and the other connects to the vacuum pump. The dressing is sealed securely in place with an occlusive dressing that extends 1¼" to 2" (3 to 5 cm) over adjacent skin all around the dressing.

Understanding VAC therapy

Vacuum-assisted closure (VAC) therapy, also called *negative-pressure wound therapy,* is an option to consider when a wound fails to heal in a timely manner. VAC therapy encourages healing by applying localized subatmospheric pressure at the site of the wound. This reduces edema and bacterial colonization and stimulates the formation of granulation tissue.

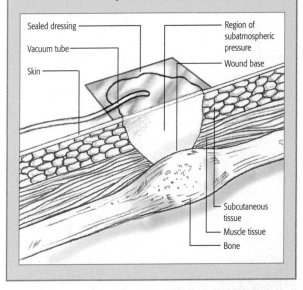

When turned on, the pump gently reduces air pressure beneath the dressing, drawing off exudate and reducing edema in surrounding tissues. This process reduces bacterial colonization, promotes granulation tissue development, increases the rate of cell mitosis, and spurs the migration of epithelial cells within the wound. Special training is required to apply the foam dressing correctly. (See *Understanding VAC therapy*.)

The large-capacity VAC device is cumbersome and isn't designed to be moved about. However, a smaller, portable version, called the *VAC Freedom* device, is available. It runs on rechargeable batteries and has a smaller drainage capacity.

The VAC Instill System allows for the automated delivery of a saline solution into the wound while still allowing for negative pressure to the wound. Patients who have infectious material or drainage in the wound benefit from the VAC Instill System. The VAC-ATS is ideal for heavily draining wounds for patients in acute care settings. This device has touch-screen operations and a 500-ml drainage capacity.

VAC therapy is useful in managing clean, slow-healing acute, subacute, or chronic exudative wounds with cavities. It's ideal for pressure ulcers or surgical wounds with depths greater than 1 cm.

The VAC device is beneficial because it:

■ cleans deeply and can manage moderate to large amounts of drainage (VAC drainage capacity is 300 ml; VAC Freedom, 300 ml; VAC Instill System, 500 ml; VAC-ATS, 500 ml)

■ has dressings that can be cut to bridge two or more wounds, or a Y-connector can be used to connect two or more wounds to one unit, permitting one VAC unit to manage multiple wounds

■ has rechargeable batteries (VAC Freedom) that last for 1 day, and is small enough to fit in pouches that can be worn at the waist or over the shoulder.

However, VAC therapy:

■ is contraindicated for use with untreated osteomyelitis, malignancies, or wounds with necrotic tissue

■ may require that the patient remain in one place or carry the unit along

- requires electricity; the VAC Freedom batteries must be recharged frequently
- can result in bruising at the wound base if used incorrectly.

WARM-UP THERAPY SYSTEM

The Warm-Up Therapy System for wounds, or noncontact normothermic wound therapy, is a temporary therapy that increases the temperature of the wound bed, thereby promoting increased blood flow in the area of the wound. The dressing in this system contains a special electronic warming card. After it's in place, the card heats to 100.4° F (38° C), bathing the wound in radiant heat. The closely sealed wound covering promotes a moist environment in the wound bed. This system is designed to remain in place for 72 hours.

The Warm-Up Therapy System may be used for acute or chronic, full- or partial-thickness wounds, regardless of etiology, that have failed to thrive with traditional therapies, including wounds with compromised blood flow, such as arterial or diabetic foot ulcers.

The wound covering can absorb a small to moderate amount of drainage.

The Warm-Up Therapy System is contraindicated for use on third-degree burns. In addition, it requires specific dressings and thorough patient teaching related to dressing changes and heat management.

Debriding agents

Debriding agents are chemical or enzyme preparations used to debride necrotic or devitalized tissues. These products are applied directly to the offending tissues in the wound. In wounds containing eschar, the eschar is crosshatched so the agent can penetrate the tissue.

Examples of debriding agents include:
- ACCUZYME
- Collagenase Santyl Ointment
- PANAFIL.

These products should be used in debriding wounds with moderate to large amounts of necrotic tissue, especially when surgical debridement isn't an option.

Debriding agents are beneficial because they:
- help control odor if they contain chlorophyll (drainage may turn green, however, and be wrongly interpreted as infection)
- require only a small amount of the agent for effective debridement.

However, debriding agents:
- may contain known allergens
- may require secondary dressings
- can cause irritation if they come in contact with surrounding skin
- can cause a burning sensation in the wound that can last for several hours
- are expensive.

Bioengineered tissue products

Bioengineered tissue products are used like skin grafts. They are meshed and placed over the entire wound bed to create a scaffold from wound edge to wound edge. This scaffolding allows the patient's own epithelial cells to migrate across the wound base more easily. (For more on bioengineered tissue products, see chapter 10, Therapeutic modalities.)

10

THERAPEUTIC MODALITIES

Therapeutic modalities have commonly been described as adjunctive modalities—treatments that are used in addition to traditional therapies. This definition is slightly outdated, however, because therapeutic modalities are now a standard of care and are central to the wound healing process. (See *How therapeutic modalities promote healing,* page 254.)

Some therapeutic modalities, such as hydrotherapy and therapeutic light, have been used since the early 1900s. Many traditional modalities are widely used in practice today, and new therapeutic modalities are always in development.

In many cases, new therapeutic modalities are based on traditional modalities. Some of the newest therapeutic modalities under development involve using near-infrared photo energy, inducing cell proliferation, and delivering ultrasound in a mist.

Selecting a treatment

Wound care needs must be considered in order to select the best treatment for the patient.

How therapeutic modalities promote healing

Various therapeutic modalities promote wound healing by:
- physically or mechanically debriding particulate and bacterial necrosis
- killing microorganisms or controlling bioburden (microorganism number)
- reducing or controlling edema and wound fluids
- increasing blood flow and tissue oxygenation
- enhancing immune or connective tissue cell function
- providing scaffolding for tissue growth.

If a wound needs debridement to remove necrosis and reduce microorganism counts, appropriate therapeutic modalities may include:
- pulsatile lavage
- whirlpool
- electrical stimulation
- laser therapy
- ultraviolet (UV) treatment (using UVC radiation)
- maggot therapy
- conservative sharp debridement.

For edema and lymphedema control and to reduce pathologic intercellular fluid loads, appropriate therapeutic modalities may include:
- electrical stimulation
- compression pumps or garments (for example, stockings).

To stimulate tissue formation by increasing blood vessel formation (angiogenesis); enhancing blood flow and the delivery of oxygen, nutrients, and immune cells; facilitating immune cell and wound bed cell function; and stimulating wound matrix formation and collagen fiber

alignment, appropriate therapeutic modalities may include:
- growth factors
- living skin equivalents
- pulsatile lavage
- UV treatment (using UVA and UVB radiation)
- ultrasound
- electrical stimulation
- laser therapy
- cell proliferation
- whirlpool.

Common therapeutic modalities

Some of the old and new therapeutic modalities widely
embraced by today's wound care practitioners are:
- biotherapy (growth factors, living skin equivalents)
- hydrotherapy (pulsatile lavage, whirlpool)
- therapeutic light (UV treatment, laser therapy)
- ultrasound
- electrical stimulation
- hyperbaric oxygen therapy (HBOT).

BIOTHERAPY
Two biotherapy methods used in wound treatment include growth factors and living skin equivalents.

Growth factors
Because of the important role that growth factors play in
the healing process (stimulating cell proliferation), they're
an important form of biotherapy.

Wound healing is a complex process that the body
undertakes to replace or repair injured tissue. Healing is
like a concert performance by an orchestra with many
musicians. When everyone knows his part and follows

the conductor, the music flows beautifully. However, if one player is out of sync with the rest of the orchestra, the result is a jumbled mixture of noise.

If various growth factors aren't synthesized, secreted, and removed from tissues with correct timing, wound healing becomes jumbled. This leaves the wound bed in a chronic state of confusion, unable to heal.

In the past decade, growth factors have been studied to determine how they function in healing and how they may be used in the treatment of chronic wounds.

Key growth factors that play roles in wound healing include:

- platelet-derived growth factor (PDGF)
- transforming growth factor beta (TGF-ß)
- basic fibroblast growth factor (bFGF)
- vascular endothelial growth factor
- insulin-like growth factor
- epidermal growth factor (EGF)

Of these growth factors, PDGF, TGF-ß, bFGF, and EGF have been through or are undergoing testing in clinical trials. At this time, the only synthetic growth factor approved for use in wound care is becaplermin (Regranex Gel 0.01%). Regranex increases wound closure by 43%. It's recommended for use on diabetic neuropathic foot ulcers that have adequate blood flow and involve tissues at and below the subcutaneous level.

Regranex can be applied to wounds using a sterile applicator, such as a swab, a tongue blade, or saline-moistened gauze. A dime-size thickness of Regranex is all that's needed. The wound can then be dressed with gauze moistened with saline.

Living skin equivalents

Another type of biotherapy available for chronic wound management involves the use of living skin equivalents.

Comparing living skin equivalents

Here's how two living skin equivalents compare.

PRODUCT	WHAT IT REPLACES	WHAT IT'S MADE FROM	WHAT IT'S USED FOR
Dermagraft	Dermis	● Human fibroblasts on a polyglactin mesh	● Burns ● Diabetic foot ulcers
Apligraf	Epidermis and dermis	● Type 1 collagen ● Human fibroblasts ● Human keratinocytes	● Venous ulcers ● Diabetic foot ulcers

Living skin equivalents are living constructs derived from biological substances, such as bovine collagen and human neonatal foreskin. Two living skin equivalents approved by the Food and Drug Administration (FDA) in the United States are Dermagraft and Graftskin (Apligraf). Dermagraft is used in treating patients with partial-thickness burns and diabetic foot ulcers. Apligraf is approved for use in both venous and diabetic foot ulcers.

All living skin equivalents should be used on wounds that are free from infection and necrosis, and have adequate blood flow to support healing. (See *Comparing living skin equivalents*.)

Dermagraft is contraindicated for use on infected wounds and wounds with sinus tracts and in individuals with known allergies to bovine products.

When applied to venous ulcers, Apligraf is used along with standard compression therapy. For a patient with diabetic foot ulcers, appropriate off-loading devices are also used.

Contraindications for Apligraf include use on wounds that are infected and use in patients with known allergies to bovine collagen or other components in the medium in which Apligraf is shipped.

HYDROTHERAPY

Hydrotherapy is one of the oldest therapeutic modalities used in wound care.

Various forms of hydrotherapy include:

- pulsatile lavage with concurrent suction
- whirlpool therapy
- jet irrigation
- irrigation with a bulb syringe or a syringe with an attached angiocatheter.

As with most treatments, the type of therapy used depends on the patient's wound type.

Pulsatile lavage

Today, most hydrotherapy treatments are delivered by pulsatile lavage. Pulsatile lavage cleans and debrides wounds by combining pulse irrigation with suction.

Advantages of using pulsatile lavage include:

- improved comfort for the patient
- mobility of the apparatus (can be performed in hospital, clinic, or home setting)
- effectiveness in reaching deep, tunneling wounds
- minimized chance of cross-contamination.

Additionally, at least one preliminary study suggests that pulsatile lavage promotes the formation of granulation tissue.

Sterile normal saline solution at room temperature is typically used for pulsatile lavage. It's applied by spray gun using a plastic, disposable fan tip. A tunneling tip is

Quantifying pressure for pulsatile lavage

The amount of pressure used for pulsatile lavage depends on the patient's wound type:
- High-impact and suction pressures are used for dirty, necrotic wounds.
- Intermediate pressures are used for infected wounds.
- Low pressures are used for clean, granulating wounds.
  Specific impact, or delivery pressures, and suction pressures are listed here.

WOUND TYPE	IMPACT PRESSURE*	SUCTION PRESSURE
Clean or granulating	4 to 6 psi	60 to 80 mm Hg
Infected	8 to 10 psi	80 to 100 mm Hg
Necrotic	10 to 12 psi	100 to 120 mm Hg

Note: Impact pressures less than 15 psi are recommended for wound management. Nurses and other staff providing wound care shouldn't exceed 15 psi of impact pressure without on-site supervision or a specific order for this pressure level.

used for deep wounds with tunnels or extensive undermining.

The solution is delivered under pressure to the wound bed and aspirated by negative pressure through a separate plastic tube in the spray gun. The therapist can control both the delivery or impact pressure of the sterile saline and the suction pressure for aspiration of the contaminated fluid. (See *Quantifying pressure for pulsatile lavage*.)

Pulsatile lavage can be used with almost any wound type: acute or chronic, large or small, infected or noninfected, and clean or necrotic.

Indications for pulsatile lavage include:
■ clean wounds—to increase granulation tissue formation

- slow-healing wounds—to increase granulation tissue formation
- infected or heavily contaminated wounds—to decrease bioburden levels
- wound bed preparation—for grafting with skin grafts or living skin equivalents
- removal of necrotic tissue or other particulate.

Currently, there are no recognized contraindications for pulsatile lavage; however, suggested precautions include:

- using lower impact and suction pressures on fragile tissue
- avoiding direct pressure over exposed nerves and blood vessels
- avoiding high-impact pressure over malignant tissue
- avoiding high-impact and suction pressures and static delivery in areas where excess suction may draw tissue into the tip as well as over grafts and exposed organs and body cavities.

Whirlpool therapy

With whirlpool therapy, part of the body is immersed in a tank of water that has been heated to a prescribed temperature and circulated by an agitator. This therapy softens tissue, removes debris and drainage, and improves blood flow to the area, enhancing the delivery of oxygen and nutrients. Treatment time is 10 to 20 minutes. A whirlpool tank may also be used for exercise therapy for patients with open wounds or when a therapeutic pool isn't available.

Whirlpool tanks are available in several sizes: small tanks for hands and feet, medium-sized tanks for lower body treatments, and large tanks for upper and lower body treatments.

Whirlpools are useful for large surface area treatments, especially when these areas are covered with tough necrotic tissue. Whirlpool treatments are useful with painful ulcers when the patient can't tolerate the pressure of a pulsatile lavage head or when allergies to local anesthetics prevent the use of pulsatile lavage.

The temperature ranges used in whirlpool therapy are:

- tepid or nonthermal—80° to 92° F (26.7° to 33.3° C)
- neutral (local skin temperature)—92° to 96° F (33.3° to 35.5° C)
- warm or thermal—96° to 104° F (35.5° to 40° C).

The appropriate water temperature depends on the patient's wound type:

- For arterial wounds, a neutral temperature is recommended with shorter treatment times (2 to 5 minutes) so that tissue metabolism isn't increased in an ischemic limb.
- Tepid whirlpool temperature and short treatment times (2 to 5 minutes) are recommended for venous ulcers because the edema associated with venous ulcers may increase with warm or hot whirlpool for extended treatments due to both heat exposure and the dependent position of the lower extremities.
- Pressure ulcers and other types of wounds can tolerate neutral to warm temperatures. Warm temperatures may inactivate the harmful enzymes in chronic wound beds.

Indications for whirlpool treatment include:

- large surface area wounds
- wounds with tough, black eschar
- wounds with particulate (such as "road rash")
- painful wounds.

Contraindications to whirlpool include:

- wound infections
- edema

- deep vein thrombosis (DVT) or acute phlebitis
- cardiovascular, pulmonary, or renal failure
- unresponsiveness or dementia
- bowel or bladder incontinence
- wounds with dry gangrene.

THERAPEUTIC LIGHT

Therapeutic light modalities include UV treatment and laser therapy.

UV treatment

Although not a form of light, UV energy or radiation is commonly categorized as therapeutic light. UV energy lies between X-rays and visible light on the electromagnetic spectrum.

UV energy has been used for more than 100 years for the treatment of slow-healing and infected wounds. Helio-therapy, or sun therapy, has most likely been used since the dawn of humankind for skin problems and other health care needs.

UV radiation is typically divided into three bands:

- UVA
- UVB
- UVC.

Here are some benefits of treatment with UVA and UVB radiation:

- Chronic pressure ulcers treated with UVA and UVB energy have exhibited increased wound healing in clinical studies.
- UVA and UVB energy enhance white blood cell (WBC) accumulation and lysosomal activity, possibly offering an explanation for UV-mediated debridement.
- UV radiation stimulates the production of interleukin-1 alpha, a cytokine that plays a role in epithelialization.

The use of UVC has been demonstrated in various wound types but is primarily used for treatment in patients with infected wounds. An added benefit of UVC is that it kills a broad spectrum of microorganisms with low exposure times and isn't likely to generate resistant microorganisms. Research has shown that UVC can kill antibiotic-resistant strains of bacteria, such as methicillin-resistant *Staphylococcus aureus*. UVC is easily administered with minimal intervention time and is inexpensive. (See *Applying UVC radiation*, page 264.)

Indications for UV treatment include:

■ chronic, slow-healing wounds
■ infected or heavily contaminated wounds
■ necrotic wounds.

Contraindications for UV treatment include certain chronic disease states, such as:

■ diabetes
■ pulmonary tuberculosis
■ hyperthyroidism
■ systemic lupus erythematosus
■ cardiac disease
■ renal disease
■ hepatic disease
■ acute eczema
■ herpes simplex.

Laser therapy

The word *laser* is actually an acronym for light amplification by stimulated emission of radiation.

Lasers can be divided into two groups:

■ Cold lasers include the helium neon, or red laser, and the gallium-arsenide laser.
■ Hot lasers encompass the carbon dioxide laser and other lasers used for surgical dissection.

Applying UVC radiation

Primarily used to treat patients with infected wounds, ultraviolet C (UVC) radiation kills a broad spectrum of microorganisms with low exposure times. Here's how it's used.

SKIN PROTECTION
First, the skin around the wound is protected with a thick application of UV-impenetrable ointment, such as zinc oxide or petrolatum. Other skin areas are covered with clean sheets. The eyes of the patient and the person administering the therapy must be covered with UV protective glasses.

EXPOSURE TIME
The UVC lamp is then placed 1″ (2.5 cm) from the wound surface and turned on for 30 to 60 seconds. This is done once daily for about 1 week or until the infection has cleared. Fungal infections may require a slightly longer treatment time (90 seconds).

DISTANCE MAINTENANCE
Tissue spacers, as shown below, may be added to maintain the appropriate distance of the lamp from the wound.

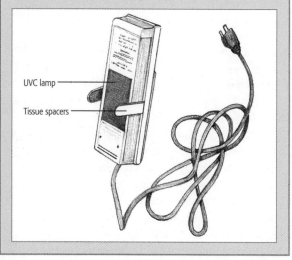

UVC lamp

Tissue spacers

In wound healing, cold lasers promote wound closure and nerve regeneration. The treatment consists of either placing the laser probe directly over selected treatment points for a specific time, according to the dose required, or using a gridlike pattern and continuously moving the probe over this grid for a specific treatment time.

Indications for laser therapy include:

- slow-healing wounds
- nerve regeneration
- pain relief.

Contraindications for laser therapy include treatments over:

- the eye
- a hemorrhage
- a malignancy
- a pregnant woman's uterus
- photosensitive skin.

ULTRASOUND

Ultrasound (mechanical pressure waves) is used to treat patients with open and closed wounds because of its non-thermal and thermal effects.

Ultrasound's thermal effects include increased blood flow to tissue, which results in increased tissue healing. Ultrasound also increases WBC migration and promotes an orderly arrangement of collagen in both open and closed wounds.

Ultrasound appears to have optimal effects when used during the inflammatory phase of wound healing. It speeds the wound's progress through the healing phases.

Ultrasound is indicated to:

- increase wound healing
- enhance blood flow
- decrease pain
- decrease inflammation.

Contraindications for ultrasound include:
- malignant tissue
- acute infections
- DVT
- ischemic areas
- plastic implants or implanted electronic devices
- irradiated areas
- treatment over the gonads, spinal cord, eyes, or a pregnant woman's uterus.

ELECTRICAL STIMULATION

Electrical stimulation is used to enhance healing of recalcitrant wounds, especially chronic pressure ulcers. The types of electrical stimulation used in wound healing include high-voltage and low-voltage pulsed current. Electrical stimulation is delivered through a device that has conductive electrodes, which are applied to the skin.

Electrical stimulation can be used to:
- orient cells
- promote cellular migration
- enhance blood flow
- increase protein synthesis and wound bed formation
- destroy microorganisms
- provide pain relief.

Electrical stimulation is indicated to:
- promote wound healing
- increase blood flow
- increase angiogenesis
- increase tissue oxygenation
- reduce wound bioburden or microbial content
- reduce pain (wound and diabetic neuropathic pain).

Contraindications for electrical stimulation include:
- malignant tissue
- untreated osteomyelitis

- treatment over pericardial area or areas related to control of cardiac and respiratory function
- treatment over some implanted electronic devices.

HYPERBARIC OXYGEN THERAPY

HBOT is the delivery of 100% oxygen through a sealed chamber.

Two forms of HBOT are used for wound healing. One form involves a total body chamber, such as that used for decompression therapy for divers, and the other involves a smaller chamber used just for the limbs. (The effectiveness of topical HBOT through small-limb chambers hasn't yet been proven through research.)

HBOT delivered by a whole body chamber increases the amount of dissolved oxygen in the blood that's available for wound healing. This increased availability of readily usable oxygen in the blood provides extra oxygen for use by cells such as neutrophils that employ oxygen-dependent processes. (The processes by which neutrophils destroy microorganisms are oxygen-based, as is cellular metabolism in general.) The increased availability of oxygen for tissues apparently relieves relative hypoxia in wounded tissues.

Evidence supporting systemic or whole body HBOT for patients with chronic wounds is evolving. Patients with venous ulcers that don't improve with traditional therapies may benefit when compression therapy is paired with systemic HBOT. Another possible use for HBOT is in patients with diabetic foot ulcers. HBOT increases nitric oxide production in the wound. Nitric oxide is a unique free radical that's important in vasodilation and neurotransmission, which play major roles in diabetic wound healing.

Indications for HBOT include:

- diabetic foot ulcers

■ venous ulcers.

　HBOT is contraindicated for patients:

■ taking antineoplastics

■ experiencing pneumothorax.

New therapeutic modalities

　Several new therapeutic modalities for wound care have evolved in the past decade. Recent developments that are new to the market or that haven't yet reached the market include:

■ monochromatic near-infrared photo energy (MIRE)

■ cell proliferation induction (CPI)

■ mist ultrasound transport therapy (MUST).

　Treatment with MIRE is U.S. FDA-approved for increasing circulation and reducing pain. The nitric oxide that's released into the bloodstream when MIRE is applied to the skin increases blood flow, delivering nutrients to the area and promoting healing. Neural function (sensation) may also improve due to increased blood flow to impaired nerves.

　CPI technology involves the use of a low-level, confined, radio frequency signal to stimulate wound healing. The signal is delivered at or near the cycle time for calcium channels, thus inducing the release of growth factors by a calcium-dependent mechanism. CPI has been shown to increase proliferation of fibroblasts and epithelial cells and has been found to stimulate wound closure in pressure wounds. CPI is still considered experimental.

　With MUST, ultrasound energy is transferred directly to the wound through a sterile saline mist. MUST enhances wound healing and decreases bacterial and necrotic debris in tissue by:

■ enhancing fibroblast migration rates (shown in the laboratory)

- increasing collagen levels (shown in an animal wound model)
- decreasing bacterial numbers (shown in both the laboratory and a patient case study)
- enhancing blood flow.

These new technologies represent a recent trend in chronic wound management—that the cells normally involved in wound healing should be stimulated as part of wound care. By doing this, cells are encouraged to do what they do best: orchestrate the complex cascade of events that lead to wound healing.

11

LEGAL AND REIMBURSEMENT ISSUES

Wounds affect thousands of people each year. They contribute to morbidity and mortality, increase the cost of health care and, sometimes, contribute to liability issues. By learning to properly evaluate wounds, you can dramatically improve the clinical and financial outcome of your wound care patient. At the same time, you'll avoid legal traps and denial of reimbursement.

An *issue* is anything questionable in provided care; it's related to some adverse occurrence or outcome.

Here are some examples of legal issues:
- a possibly negligent action or omission by a health care provider
- deviation from an accepted standard of care
- inconsistencies in documentation.

A common question that arises in issues of medical malpractice is "Has the practitioner met accepted standards of care?" For example, did a wound care specialist fail to implement preventive measures even though a patient was identified as being at risk for pressure ulcers?

Standards of care

To safeguard your practice, get to know what standards you're held to in the event of a legal issue.

Standard of care is a term used to specify what's reasonable under a certain set of circumstances. Standards are used to define certain aspects of a profession, such as the:

- focus of its pursuits
- beneficiaries of service
- responsibilities of its practitioners.

In health care, the prevailing professional standard of care is defined as the level of care, skill, and treatment deemed acceptable and appropriate by similar health care providers. A standard is a yardstick against which effective care can be measured.

The standards for wound care practice are derived from several sources:

- Agency for Healthcare Research and Quality (AHRQ) guidelines
- Patient Care Partnership
- facility- and unit-specific policies and procedures
- job descriptions (see *How job descriptions help to set standards of care,* page 272)
- American Nurses Association (ANA) Standards of Clinical Nursing Practice
- state nurse practice acts and guidelines.

AGENCY FOR HEALTHCARE RESEARCH AND QUALITY GUIDELINES

Guidelines from the AHRQ—formerly the Agency for Health Care Policy and Research, or AHCPR—are a primary source of wound care standards for all health care practitioners.

How job descriptions help to set standard of care

How does your employer define the health care team's roles and relationships? Depending on the practice setting—such as hospital, home, or extended care facility—your role may vary.

To protect patients and staff members, firm practice guidelines are needed for all personnel to make sure that job descriptions are accurate. If health care employees practice outside their formal job descriptions, the facility's legal counsel or the insurance company could win a judgment against those employees to recover some of the losses incurred. Carrying personal malpractice insurance is usually recommended to protect the practitioner.

The AHRQ supports research and provides evidence-based information related to health care. (See *Spotlight on the AHRQ*.)

In the past decade, several campaigns have focused on establishing and publishing best practice guidelines for the prevention and treatment of pressure ulcers. In the 1990s, the AHRQ sponsored the *Clinical Practice Guidelines* for effective and appropriate care of specific patient populations. Two are specific to wound care:

■ *Prevention of Pressure Ulcers* (AHCPR *Clinical Practice Guideline* number 3) deals with tools to identify patients at risk for developing pressure ulcers and guidelines for basic preventive skin care and early treatment.

■ *Treatment of Pressure Ulcers* (AHCPR *Clinical Practice Guideline* number 15) provides specific aspects of pressure ulcer care and corresponding evidence to support each recommendation.

PATIENT CARE PARTNERSHIP

The *Patient Care Partnership*, formerly the *Patient's Bill of Rights*, is another recognized basis for standards of care.

Spotlight on the AHRQ

The Agency for Healthcare Research and Quality is a federal agency that sponsors and conducts research on major areas of health care, including:
- quality improvement and patient safety
- outcomes and effectiveness of care
- clinical practice and technology assessment
- health care organization and delivery systems
- health care costs and sources of payment.

The American Hospital Association first sanctioned a *Patient's Bill of Rights* in 1973 to establish standards of treatment that each patient can expect, including:
- the right to considerate and respectful care
- the right to know, by name, the practitioner accountable for his care and to acquire from the practitioner thorough information related to his diagnosis, treatment, and prognosis
- the right to receive enough information to give informed consent
- the right to refuse treatment
- the right to privacy relative to his medical care
- the right to confidentiality
- the right to solicit hospital services even if it means evaluation and referral to an accepting hospital
- the right to acquire information such as the names of individuals involved in providing his care and whether they are students, residents, or trainees
- the right to be informed if the hospital plans to engage in experimental treatment and the right to refuse to partake in such treatment
- the right to expect follow-up care on discharge
- the right to review and receive an explanation of his bill

■ the right to understand hospital rules and regulations
related to patient conduct.

FACILITY- AND UNIT-SPECIFIC POLICIES AND PROCEDURES

The policies and procedures in your facility are also used
to establish standards of care.

Policies and procedures are commonly used in litigation claims. Too often, practitioners are informed of policies and procedures but don't take time to examine and
understand them. Deviating from facility policies and procedures suggests failure to meet the facility's standards of
care.

STANDARDS OF CLINICAL NURSING PRACTICE

For professional nursing, the *Standards of Clinical Nursing
Practice* outlines the expectancy of the comprehensive
professional role within which all nurses must practice.
Nursing practice standards ensure that the quality of
nursing care, documentation, consistency, accountability,
and professional credibility are upheld.

The ANA first published the *Standards of Nursing
Practice* in 1973. Since then, specialty nursing organizations have developed their own standards of practice in
various areas of nursing, such as in emergency, periopera-
tive, oncologic, and critical care nursing. Some of these
standards were developed and published in collaboration
with the ANA.

In 1991, the *Standards of Nursing Practice* was revised
with participation from state nurses associations and specialty nursing organizations. The revised publication—
Standards of Clinical Nursing Practice—is a comprehensive
outline of expectations for all nurses. *Standards of Clinical
Nursing Practice* is composed of authoritative statements

Learning about wound care organizations

In addition to the WOCN, there are several other professional organizations related to wound care:

- American Academy of Wound Management
- Wound Care Education Institute
- National Alliance of Wound Care
- Association for Advancement of Wound Care
- Wound Healing Society.

describing a level of care or performance common to all nurses. It sets a standard by which the quality of nursing practice can be judged.

The Wound, Ostomy, and Continence Nurses Society (WOCN) is the professional organization for wound, ostomy, and continence (WOC) nurses (formerly known as *enterostomal nurses*). WOC nurses are experts in skin care and wound management. In 1987, the WOCN standards of care were developed for patients with dermal wounds (pressure sores and leg ulcers). Since then, the standards have been revised to reflect advances in technology and updated research findings.

In addition to the WOCN, there are several other professional organizations related to wound care. (See *Learning about wound care organizations*.)

STATE NURSE PRACTICE ACTS AND GUIDELINES

Nurse practice acts and guidelines set by each state are also used to establish standards of care for nurses.

State nurse practice acts are laws that define which treatments, actions, and functions can be performed or delegated in each state.

For example, conservative sharp debridement is a method of removing loose, nonviable tissue with sterile instruments. According to most state nurse practice acts, it may be performed by "trained health care professionals" such as registered nurses but would be beyond the scope of practice for licensed practical nurses. It's each nurse's professional responsibility to understand her scope of practice. If a nurse is licensed in more than one state, she needs to make sure that she's familiar with the specific guidelines of the state in which she's practicing.

Litigation

Litigation is a lawsuit that's contested in court to enforce a right or pursue a resolution. Examples of legal liability specifically related to wound care usually involve claims of negligence, such as:
▪ failure to prevent
▪ failure to treat
▪ failure to heal.

Negligence, which is now recognized as a form of malpractice, is defined as failure to meet a standard of care—in other words, failure to do what another reasonably prudent health care provider would do in similar circumstances.

Practitioners are being sued individually for malpractice with increasing frequency. Malpractice is a health care professional's wrongful conduct, improper discharge of professional duties, or failure to meet standards of care that result in harm to another person. Most malpractice litigation comes as a result of claims that a health care provider failed to:
▪ provide physical protection
▪ monitor or assess
▪ promptly respond

■ properly administer a drug.

Practitioners in critical care, emergency, trauma, and obstetrics and those who practice as specialists are most vulnerable.

Four criteria must be verified to determine whether a medical malpractice claim is merited:

■ A *duty* must be established with the patient. What this means is that the practitioner accepts accountability for the care and treatment of the patient.

■ A *breach of duty or of standard of care* by the practitioner must be determined to evaluate whether there has been an act of negligence or breach of duty that resulted in harm to the patient.

■ *Proximate cause* or *causal connection* must be established between the breach of duty or standard of care and the damages or injuries to the patient. The patient must prove that damages were due directly to the practitioner's negligence and that the damages were foreseeable. In other words, were the damages a direct result of the negligence?

■ *Damages,* or *injuries,* to the patient must be presented as evidence as a result of the alleged negligence. These damages can be physical (disfigurement or pain and suffering), mental (mental anguish), or financial (past, present, or future medical expenses).

If the patient-plaintiff can establish these four components, malpractice litigation is merited.

AVOIDING LITIGATION

The key to reducing your risk of involvement in malpractice litigation is prevention. However, even if you provide optimum care to every patient, there's no guarantee that your actions will never be called into question in a litigation case. If that happens, you must be aware of how you're protected.

Many practitioners practice under the perception that they're protected by their facility's or employer's insurance policy. In most legal claims, your interests and the interests of your employer are comparable. However, the insurance company that provides your employer's coverage may be more allegiant to the employer than to you. In addition, the employer's insurance may not cover you if your performance fell outside your job description or if you didn't follow written policy and procedure.

Practicing without your own malpractice insurance is risky. Malpractice insurance doesn't keep you from getting sued, but it may lift most of the financial burden and fear of a lawsuit off your shoulders. Remember, it's expensive to prove your innocence.

Excellent documentation is the key to minimizing your liability. It's direct evidence of your evaluation and care related to wounds. The medical record is your best protection and first line of defense. (See *Documentation do's and don'ts*.)

A patient's satisfaction with care also reduces liability. Typically, a malpractice claim represents the connection between patient injury and patient anger. Good communication with the patient and his family is essential to maintaining a good connection.

Health care is a service industry, so you need to incorporate good customer service into your daily practice, including:

- being respectful and courteous; people become angry when treated rudely
- being attentive; give patients the time that they need
- being sympathetic and empathetic; concern pays off in the long run
- being considerate and honest; patients recognize honesty, which makes them feel better about the care they receive

Documentation do's and don'ts

To protect yourself against liability, document as accurately as possible by following these guidelines.

DO
● Chart factually, specifically, and concisely. Present your observations and interventions clearly and concisely.
● Chart thoroughly; malpractice claims are commonly filed years later, and the passage of time impairs your ability to remember details.
● Chart promptly. Making tardy or late entries may lead to inadvertent omissions.

DON'T
● Chart personal observations, opinions, feelings, or beliefs. These aspects of care are irrelevant.

■ recognizing your limits; ask for help or a second opinion if you have doubts
■ staying current; continuing education is a professional responsibility.

Reimbursement

Understanding finances as they relate to wound care is essential when you're providing care to high-risk patients and those with alterations in skin integrity, such as an ulcer or a wound. Why? Because treating wounds can be costly.

With the ever-increasing costs of health care, it's important to recognize your role when it comes to reimbursement. Putting cost-effective wound care into clinical practice requires knowledge of payment systems and documentation strategies.

PAYMENT SYSTEMS

The language of health insurance is complicated; make sure you can recognize basic terms related to payment systems.

Examples of payment systems include:

- Medicare
- Medicaid
- managed care
- private pay.

Medicare

Medicare is a federal insurance program for people age 65 and older, specific disabled individuals, and people with diagnosed end-stage renal disease. It's administered by the Centers for Medicare and Medicaid Services (CMS).

Medicare is split into Part A (hospital insurance), Part B (medical insurance), and Part D (drug insurance):

- Part A coverage encompasses inpatient hospital care, inpatient skilled nursing facility care associated with inpatient hospitalization, home health care after inpatient hospitalization, and hospice care.
- Part B coverage includes services provided by doctors and other health care professionals, ambulance services, and durable medical supplies and equipment (such as wound care dressings and other supplies).
- Part D coverage includes medications for anyone covered by Medicare Part A or B. There are several different plans for the patient to choose from. Enrollment is voluntary.

CMS contracts with insurance companies to process and pay claims for health care provided to Medicare beneficiaries. Payment for services and products varies according to practice settings, such as acute care hospitals, skilled nursing facilities, home health care agencies, outpatient facilities, and hospices.

Claims for services and products are submitted using a coding system known as the Healthcare Common Procedure Coding System, or HCPCS. Current Procedural Terminology codes, which are commonly called *CPT codes,* are used to bill services.

Medicaid

Medicaid is a medical assistance program for indigent individuals who are elderly, blind, or disabled and for needy families with dependent children. Although cojointly funded through federal and state regulations, it's administered by state agencies. Reimbursement guidelines vary for each state and in each practice setting.

Managed care

Managed care is a health insurance program that combines benefits presented through Medicare and Medicare Plus Choice (Medicare Part C). Medicare Plus Choice combines Medicare and private insurance programs— such as health maintenance organizations and preferred provider organizations programs—that may provide benefits not covered by Medicare. Reimbursement is based on fee structures established by each program.

Private pay

Private insurance reimbursement and benefits are also provided in a variety of ways. Like the other programs, they have established contracts to pay for services furnished by providers based on reasonable charges. Reasonable charges may include whatever is considered necessary to provide services related to patient care.

DOCUMENTATION STRATEGIES

Health insurance payers are directly involved in treatment decisions because they make decisions regarding payment for medical services and supplies. The fact is most denials of reimbursement result from insufficient or inconsistent documentation.

Assessment and documentation are used to determine the patient's care plan and reimbursement decisions. The information used in making care plan and payment decisions come from the data you provide. Make sure your documentation:

- clearly supports the clinical assessment
- accurately recounts a succession of outcomes related to patient care
- supports payment.

Outcome tracking and reevaluation of the care plan are used to track the healing of a patient's wound. They must be done to avoid reimbursement denial. To maximize reimbursement, the practitioner must properly stage and assess wounds and document the patient's progress. Third-party payers no longer pay for continuous wound treatment. They want to see evidence of progress and healing.

Pressure ulcer prediction and prevention algorithm

This algorithm, developed by the Agency for Healthcare Policy and Research (now the Agency for Healthcare Research and Quality), can be used to identify patients at risk for pressure ulcers and to prevent pressure ulcer formation. For detailed guidelines, refer to the Clinical Practice Guidelines available online at *www.ahrq.gov/*.

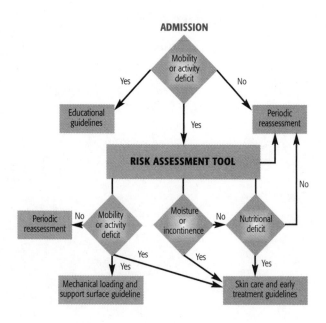

Source: "Pressure Ulcers in Adults: Prediction and Prevention," Clinical Practice Guideline Number 3. AHCPR Publication No. 92-0047. Rockville, Md.: Agency for Health Care Policy and Research, Public Health Service, U.S. Department of Health and Human Services, May 1992.

Pressure ulcer management algorithm

This algorithm, developed by the Agency for Healthcare Policy and Research (now the Agency for Healthcare Research and Quality), can be used to outline the treatment plan for a patient who has a pressure ulcer. For detailed guidelines, refer to the Clinical Practice Guidelines available online at *www.ahrq.gov/*.

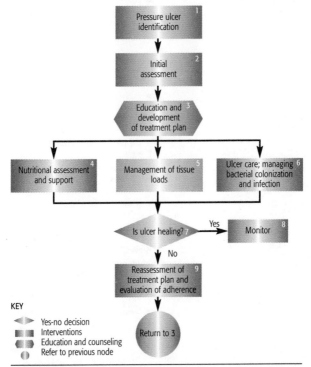

Source: "Pressure Ulcer Treatment," Clinical Practice Guideline Number 3. AHCPR Publication No. 95-0652. Rockville, Md.: Agency for Health Care Policy and Research, Public Health Service, U.S. Department of Health and Human Services, 1992.

Quick guide to wound care dressings

DRESSING TYPE	INDICATIONS	PRODUCTS
Alginate	• Wounds with moderate to heavy drainage • Wounds with tunneling	• AlgiCell Calcium Alginate • AlgiDERM Calcium Alginate Dressing or Packing • AlgiSite M • CarboFlex Odor Control Dressing • CarraGinate High G Calcium Alginate Wound Dressing with Acemannan Hydrogel • CarraSorb H Calcium Alginate Wound Dressing • Comfeel Seasorb • Curasorb • Curasorb Zinc • DermaGinate • Hyperion Advanced Alginate Dressing • KALGINATE Calcium Alginate Wound Dressing • KALTOSTAT Wound Dressing • Maxorb CMC/Alginate Dressing • Melgisorb • Restore CalciCare Wound Care Dressing • Sorbsan Topical Wound Dressing • 3M Tegagen HI and HG Alginate Dressings
Biological	• Temporary dressing for skin graft donor sites and burns	• Hyalofill Biopolymeric Wound Dressing • Inerpan Temporary Wound Dressing • Oasis Wound Dressing • Silon Wound Dressing
Collagen	• Chronic, nonhealing, granulated wound beds • Wounds with tunneling	• FIBRACOL PLUS Collagen Wound Dressing with Alginate • Kollagen-Medifil Pads • Kollagen-SkinTemp Sheets

DRESSING TYPE	INDICATIONS	PRODUCTS
Composite	• Primary or secondary dressing on wounds with light to moderate drainage • Protection for peripheral and central I.V. lines	• Alldress • CompDress Island Dressing • COVADERM PLUS • DuDress Film Top Island Dressing • MPM Multi-Layered Dressing • Repel Wound Dressing • Stratasorb • TELFA Adhesive Dressing • Telfa Island Dressing • TELFA PLUS Island Dressing • 3M Medipore+Pad Soft Cloth Adhesive Wound Dressing • 3M Tegaderm+Pad Transparent Dressing with Absorbent Pad • Viasorb Wound Dressing
Contact layer	• Wounds with minimal, moderate, and heavy drainage; allows for flow of drainage to a secondary dressing while preventing dressing from adhering to the wound	• Conformant 2 Wound Veil • DERMANET Wound Contact Layer • Mepitel • N-TERFACE Interpositional Surfacing Material • Profore Wound Contact Layer • Telfa Clear • 3M Tegapore Wound Contact Material • VersaDress Wound Contact Layer
Foam	• Primary or secondary dressing on wounds with minimal to moderate drainage (including around tubes) when a nonadherent surface is important	• Allevyn and Allevyn Adhesive Hydrophilic Polyurethane Foam Dressing • Allevyn Cavity Wound Dressing • Biatain Adhesive Foam Dressing • Biatain Non-Adhesive Foam Dressing • CarraSmart Foam Dressing • Curafoam Plus Foam Dressing • Curafoam Wound Dressing • EPIGARD • Flexzan Topical Wound Dressing • Hydrasorb Foam Wound Dressing • HydroCell Adhesive Foam Dressing • HydroCell Foam Dressing • HydroCell Thin Adhesive Foam Dressing • LO PROFILE FOAM Wound Dressing • Lyofoam A Polyurethane Foam Dressing

DRESSING TYPE	INDICATIONS	PRODUCTS
Foam *(continued)*		• Lyofoam C Polyurethane Foam Dressing with Activated Carbon • Lyofoam Extra Polyurethane Foam Dressing • Lyofoam Polyurethane Foam Dressing • Lyofoam T Polyurethane Foam Dressing • Mepilex • Mepilex Border • Mitraflex • Mitraflex Plus • Odor-Absorbent Dressing • Optifoam Adhesive Foam Island Dressing • Optifoam Non-Adhesive Foam Island Dressing • POLYDERM BORDER Hydrophilic Polyurethane Foam Dressing • Polyderm Hydrophilic Polyurethane Foam Dressing • Polyderm Plus Barrier Foam Dressing • PolyMem Adhesive Cloth Dressings • PolyMem Adhesive Film Dressings • PolyMem Calcium Alginate • PolyMem Non-Adhesive Dressings • PolyTube Tube-Site Dressing • PolyWic Cavity Wound Filler • SOF-FOAM Dressing • SorbaCell Foam Dressing • TIELLE Hydropolymer Adhesive Dressing • TIELLE PLUS Hydropolymer Dressing • VigiFOAM Dressing
Hydrocolloid	• Wounds with minimal to moderate drainage, including wounds with necrosis or slough • Secondary dressings (sheet dressings)	• CarraSmart Hydrocolloid with Acemannan Hydrogel • CombiDERM ACD Absorbent Cover Dressing • CombiDERM Non-Adhesive • Comfeel Paste and Powder • Comfeel Plus Contour Dressing • Comfeel Plus Pressure Relief Dressing • Comfeel Plus Triangle Dressing

DRESSING TYPE	**INDICATIONS**	**PRODUCTS**
Hydrocolloid *(continued)*		• Comfeel Plus Ulcer Dressing • Comfeel TRIAD Hydrophilic Wound Dressing • DermaFilm HD • DermaFilm Thin • DERMATELL • DERMATELL SECURE • DuoDERM CGF • DuoDERM CGF Border • DuoDERM Extra Thin • DuoDERM Hydroactive Paste • Exuderm • Exuderm LP • Exuderm RCD • Exuderm Sacrum • Exuderm Ultra • Hydrocol • Hydrocol Sacral • Hydrocol Thin • Hyperion Hydrocolloid Dressing • MPM Excel Hydrocolloid Wound Dressing • PrimaCol Bordered Hydrocolloid Wound Dressing • PrimaCol Hydrocolloid Dressing • PrimaCol Specialty Hydrocolloid Dressing • PrimaCol Thin Hydrocolloid Dressing • Procol Hydrocolloid Dressing • RepliCare • RepliCare Thin • Restore Cx Wound Care Dressing • Restore Extra Thin Dressing • Restore Plus Wound Care Dressing • Restore Wound Care Dressing • SignaDRESS Hydrocolloid Dressing • Sorbex • Sorbexthin • 3M Tegasorb Hydrocolloid Dressings • 3M Tegasorb THIN Hydrocolloid Dressings • Ulcer Care Dressing • Ultec Hydrocolloid Dressing • Ultec Pro Alginate Hydrocolloid Dressing

DRESSING TYPE	INDICATIONS	PRODUCTS
Hydrogel	• Dry wounds • Wounds with minimal drainage • Wounds with necrosis	• AcryDerm Moist Hydrophilic Wound Dressing • Amerigel Ointment • Aquaflo • AquaGauze Hydrogel Impregnated Gauze Dressing • Aquasite Amorphous Hydrogel • Aquasite Impregnated Gauze Hydrogel • Aquasite Impregnated Non-Woven Hydrogel • Aquasite Sheet Hydrogel • Aquasorb Hydrogel Wound Dressing • Bandage Roll with ClearSite • Biolex Wound Gel • CarraDres Clear Hydrogel Sheet • CarraGauze Pads and Strips with Acemannan Hydrogel • CarraSmart Gel Wound Dressing with Acemannan Hydrogel • Carrasyn Gel Wound Dressing with Acemannan Hydrogel • Carrasyn Spray Gel Wound Dressing with Acemannan Hydrogel • Carrasyn V with Acemannan Hydrogel • Comfort-Aid • Curafil Gel Wound Dressing and Impregnated Strips • Curagel • CURASOL Gel Wound Dressing • DermaGel Hydrogel Sheet • Dermagran Hydrophilic Wound Dressing • Dermagran Zinc-Saline Hydrogel • DermaSyn • DiaB Gel with Acemannan Hydrogel • Elasto-Gel • Elasto-Gel Plus • Elta Hydrogel Impregnated Gauze • Elta Hydrovase Wound Gel • Elta Wound Gel • FlexiGel • Gentell Hydrogel • Hypergel

DRESSING TYPE	INDICATIONS	PRODUCTS
Hydrogel *(continued)*		• Hyperion Hydrogel Gauze Dressing • Hyperion Hydrophilic Wound Dressing • Hyperion Hydrophilic Wound Gel • Iamin Hydrating Gel • IntraSite Gel • MPM Excel Gel • MPM GelPad Hydrogel Saturated Dressing • MPM Regenecare • Normlgel • NU-GEL Collagen Wound Gel • PanoGauze Hydrogel Impregnated Gauze Dressing • PanoPlex Hydrogel Wound Dressing • Phyto Derma Wound Gel • Purilon Gel • RadiaGel with Acemannan Hydrogel • RadiaDres Gel Sheet with Acemannan Hydrogel • Restore Hydrogel Dressing • SAF-Gel Hydrating Dermal Wound Dressing • Skintegrity Amorphous Hydrogel • Skintegrity Hydrogel Impregnated Gauze • SoloSite Gel Conformable Wound Dressing • SoloSite Wound Gel • TenderWet Gel Pad • 3M Tegagel Hydrogel Wound Fillers • TOE-AID Toe and Nail Dressing • Ultrex Gel Wound Dressing • Vigilon Primary Wound Dressing • Wound Dressing with ClearSite • WOUN'DRES Collagen Hydrogel
Specialty absorptive	• Infected or noninfected wounds with heavy drainage	• AQUACEL • BAND-AID Brand Island Surgical Dressings • BreakAway Wound Dressing • CombiDERM ACD Absorbent Cover Dressing • CombiDERM Non-Adhesive • Covaderm Adhesive Wound Dressing

DRESSING TYPE	INDICATIONS	PRODUCTS
Specialty absorptive *(continued)*		• CURITY Abdominal Pads • DuPad Abdominal Pads, Open End • DuPad Abdominal Pads, Sealed End • EXU-DRY • Mepore • Multipad Non-Adherent Wound Dressing • Primapore Specialty Absorptive Dressing • Sofsorb Wound Dressing • SURGI-PAD Combine Dressing • TENDERSORB WET-PRUF Abdominal Pads
Transparent film	• Partial-thickness wounds with minimal exudate • Wounds with eschar	• BIOCLUSIVE Select Transparent Dressing • BIOCLUSIVE Transparent Dressing • Blisterfilm • CarraFilm Transparent Film Dressing • CarraSmart Film Transparent Film Dressing • ClearCell Transparent Film Dressing • ClearSite Transparent Membrane • DermaView • Mefilm • OpSite • OpSite FLEXIGRID • OpSite PLUS • OpSite Post-Op • Polyskin II Transparent Dressing • Polyskin MR Moisture Responsive Transparent Dressing • ProCyte Transparent Film Dressing • Suresite • 3M Tegaderm HP Transparent Dressing • Transeal Transparent Wound Dressing • UniFlex

DRESSING TYPE	INDICATIONS	PRODUCTS
Wound filler	● Primary dressing on an infected or a noninfected wound with minimal to moderate drainage that requires packing	● AcryDerm STRANDS Absorbent Wound Filler ● Bard Absorption Dressing ● CarraSorb M Freeze Dried Gel Wound Dressing with Acemannan Hydrogel ● Catrix Wound Dressing ● Catrix 5 Rejuvenation Cream ● Catrix 10 Ointment ● FlexiGel Strands Absorbent Wound Dressing ● hyCURE ● hyCURE SMART GEL ● IODOFLEX PAD ● IODOSORB GEL ● Kollagen-Medifil II Gel ● Kollagen-Medifil II Particles ● Multidex Maltodextrin Wound Dressing Gel or Powder

Wound and skin documentation tool

When performing wound and skin care, a pictorial demonstration is often helpful to identify the wound site or sites. Using the wound and skin documentation tool here, the practitioner identifies that the left second toe has a red, partial-thickness, vascular ulcer.

PATIENT'S NAME (LAST, MIDDLE, FIRST)		ATTENDING PHYSICIAN		ROOM NUMBER	ID NUMBER
Johnson, Ruth		Dr. T. Marshall		123-2	01726

WOUND ASSESSMENT:

NUMBER	1	2	3	4	5	6
DATE	1/08/07					
TIME	1330					
LOCATION	ⓛ second toe					
STAGE	II					
APPEARANCE	G					
SIZE-LENGTH	0.5 cm					
SIZE-WIDTH	1 cm					
COLOR/FLR.	RD					
DRAINAGE	0					
ODOR	0					
VOLUME	0					
INFLAMMATION	0					
SIZE INFLAM.						

KEY

Stage:
    I. Red or discolored
    II. Skin break/blister
    III. Subcutaneous tissue
    IV. Muscle and/or bone

Appearance:
    D = Depth
    E = Eschar
    G = Granulation
    IN = Inflammation
    NEC = Necrotic
    PK = Pink
    SL = Slough
    TN = Tunneling
    UND = Undermining
    MX = Mixed (specify)

Color of Wound
Floor:
    RD = Red
    Y = Yellow
    BLK = Black
    MX = Mixed (specify)

Drainage:
    0 = None
    SR = Serous
    SS = Serosanguineous
    BL = Blood
    PR = Purulent

Odor:
    0 = None
    MLD = Mild
    FL = Foul

Volume:
    0 = None
    SC = Scant
    MOD = Moderate
    LG = Large

Inflammation:
    0 = None
    PK = Pink
    RD = Red

WOUND ANATOMICAL LOCATION:
(circle affected area)

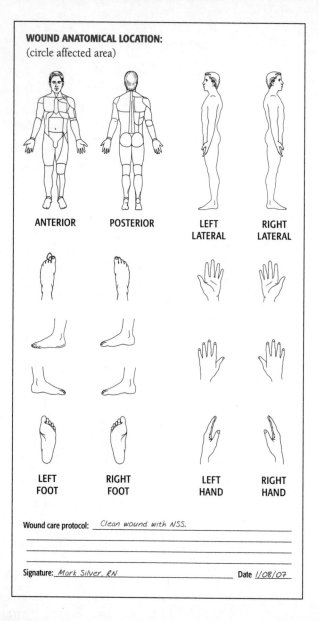

ANTERIOR   POSTERIOR   LEFT
                                 LATERAL   RIGHT
                                                LATERAL

LEFT   RIGHT   LEFT
FOOT   FOOT   HAND   RIGHT
                                                HAND

Wound care protocol: _Clean wound with NSS._

Signature: _Mark Silver, RN_   Date _1/08/07_

Selected references

Bale, S., and Jones, V. *Wound Care Nursing*, 2nd ed. St. Louis: Elsevier Mosby Ltd, 2006.

Baxter, H. "How a Discipline Came of Age: A History of Wound Care," *Journal of Wound Care* 11(10):383-86, 388, 390, November 2002.

Bryant, R., and Nix, D. *Acute and Chronic Wounds*. St. Louis: Elsevier Mosby, 2007.

Butter, A., et al, "Vacuum-Assisted Closure for Wound Management in the Pediatric Population," *Journal of Pediatric Surgery* 41(5):940-42, May 2006.

Frykberg, R. "A Summary of Guidelines for Managing the Diabetic Foot," *Advances in Skin & Wound Care* 18(4):209-14, May 2005.

Helberg, D., et al. "Treatment of Pressure Ulcers: Results of a Study Comparing Evidence and Practice," *Ostomy Wound Management* 52(8):60-72, August 2006.

Hess, C.T. *Clinical Guide to Wound Care,* 5th ed. Philadelphia: Lippincott Williams & Wilkins, 2005.

Irion, G., et al. "Accelerated Closure of Biopsy-Type Wounds by Mechanical Stimulation," *Advances in Skin & Wound Care* 19(2):97-102, March 2006.

Langemo, D., et al. "Nutritional Considerations in Wound Care," *Advances in Skin & Wound Care* 19(6):297-303, July-August 2006.

McNees, P. "Skin and Wound Assessment and Care in Oncology," *Seminars in Oncology Nursing* 22(3):130-43, August 2006.

Pieper, B. *Wound Care: An Issue of Nursing Clinics*. Philadelphia: Elsevier Saunders, 2005.

Skillmasters: Wound Care. Philadelphia: Lippincott Williams & Wilkins, 2007.

Thompson, C., and Fuhrman, M.P. "Nutrients and Wound Healing: Still Searching for the Magic Bullet," *Nutrition Clinical Practice* 20(3):331-47, 2005.

Index

i refers to an illustration; t refers to a table.

---

i refers to an illustration; t refers to a table.

i refers to an illustration; t refers to a table.

i refers to an illustration; t refers to a table.

---

i refers to an illustration; t refers to a table.

i refers to an illustration; t refers to a table.

---

i refers to an illustration; t refers to a table.

No Newer ed. dm 2/17/14